YOUR KIDS
AT RISK

DI018276

YOUR KIDS AT RISK

HOW TEEN SEX THREATENS OUR SONS AND DAUGHTERS

MEG MEEKER, M.D.

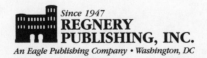

Since 1947
REGNERY
PUBLISHING, INC.
An Eagle Publishing Company • Washington, DC

Copyright © 2007 Meg Meeker

All rights reserved. No part of this publication may be reproduced or transmitted in any form or by any means electronic or mechanical, including photocopy, recording, or any information storage and retrieval system now known or to be invented, without permission in writing from the publisher, except by a reviewer who wishes to quote brief passages in connection with a review written for inclusion in a magazine, newspaper, or broadcast.

Cataloging-in-Publication Data on file with the Library of Congress
ISBN 978-1-59698-513-1

Published in the United States by
Regnery Publishing Company
One Massachusetts Avenue, NW
Washington, DC 20001

www.regnery.com

Hardcover edition published under the title *Epidemic*
First paperback edition published in 2007

Manufactured in the United States of America

10 9 8 7 6 5 4 3 2 1

Books are available in quantity for promotional or premium use. Write to Director of Special Sales, Regnery Publishing, Inc., One Massachusetts Avenue, NW, Washington, DC 20001, for information on discounts and terms or call (202) 216-0600.

The information contained in this book is not a substitute for medical counseling and care. All matters pertaining to your physical health should be supervised by a health care professional.

Author's Disclaimer: As you read this book, you'll meet many of my young patients for whom STDs and sex have dramatically altered their lives. I have significantly changed the names, situations, and ages of my patients in order to protect their privacy. You will read collages of their lives strung together by real medical situations which I have encountered during the past 20 years of my practice. But the medical, psychological, and family problems are all too real, and the medical diagnoses and situations are accurate.

To the love of my life, my husband, Walt
And to the joys in my life, Mary,
Charlotte, Laura, and Walter

Contents

Sponge ▪ Sex Is Big ▪ Sex Symbols as Role Models ▪ Cool People Are Promiscuous ▪ So What Are Parents to Do?

NINE High-Risk Sex   147

Why It's Happening ▪ Oral Sex: A Craze with Consequences ▪ Oral Sex Is No Protection ▪ Mary Ellen's Story ▪ Homosexual Sexual Activity ▪ Multiple Partners ▪ Can I Watch? Voyeurism ▪ Everything But Sex... ▪ Sex, Drugs, and Alcohol ▪ Jared's Story ▪ The Alcohol-Disease Connection ▪ Cybersex ▪ Good Sex/Bad Sex

PART III: WHAT TO KNOW, WHAT TO DO

TEN Adolescent in Body and Mind   175

When Puberty Strikes ▪ Andrea's Story ▪ STDs and the Adolescent Girl's Body ▪ When Boys Reach Puberty ▪ Sex and Sexuality ▪ Emancipation ▪ Identity Formation ▪ Inability To Think in the Abstract

ELEVEN Connectedness   197

Our Teenagers Want Connectedness with Us ▪ Developing Great Relationships with Our Teens ▪ Connecting Through Communication ▪ Connecting Through Intimacy ▪ The Magic Touch ▪ Connecting Through Emotional Intimacy ▪ Connecting Through Love ▪ Connecting Through Appreciation ▪ Parental Disapproval of Sex

TWELVE Holding Off   215

Teaching Kids to Postpone Sex ▪ Ambivalence Is Permission ▪ It's Never Too Late ▪ In Conclusion

Introduction to the 2007 Edition

I have a very peculiar job. I am a pediatrician who talks to a lot of kids about an enormous problem many parents and professionals don't want to see—let alone discuss openly. I talk about the explosive epidemic of sexually transmitted infections threatening kids. Some compare my profession to that of a veterinarian—one who diagnoses illnesses in patients who can't (or won't) talk. Others, after they have listened to my lectures, think that I am an obstetrician/gynecologist. I have even gotten letters from folks who think that I am a psychiatrist. I am none of these things. I am a pediatrician and a mother who has seen too much pain in too many kids. Please let this sink in for a moment: I am a pediatrician talking about sexually transmitted infections. That alone is a sobering reality.

In the mid-1980s, I completed my pediatric residency training in a large inner-city pediatric hospital. I cared for babies of teens and for the teens themselves. I cried a lot during those years because I saw enormous pain in the eyes of these child mothers. But I took comfort in the thought that perhaps the bulk of the pain was isolated in the inner city, in kids who awoke every day to a single mom who drank too much or to a filthy, overcrowded apartment.

After six years of treating kids with sexually transmitted infections, I told my husband that it was time to move on. I wanted to treat plump, full-term babies whose mothers read child-care books and researched the safest toys.

I wanted to leave behind my clinical portion of the 19 million new sexually transmitted diseases that occur in Americans every year. Burn that number—*19 million*—into your mind. That's *new cases, every year*. I wanted no part of them any longer. I was tired.

We moved to the suburbs and I cared for my friends' kids and my kids' friends. I was relieved that the mess was far away, locked in pockets of troubled, high-risk kids who needed quality medical care from a fresh crew of physicians.

What occurred in my medical practice over the following ten-plus years shook me to the core. Slowly, meticulously, those wretched infections surfaced in the bodies of my new crop of patients. I was angry and sad. These kids were not "high-risk" according to the medical literature. They had stable homes, clean clothes, and attended excellent schools. Chlamydia and herpes weren't supposed to be here.

In my optimism, I hoped that my experience was unusual. So I turned to the medical literature to find out what was happening around the country. What I found rattled me. On my (and your) watch, an epidemic had exploded among our kids. From 1960 to 2000 the number of sexually transmitted diseases in our children skyrocketed. I asked my colleagues in internal medicine, pediatrics, and family practice if they were aware of the numbers I showed them. They shook their heads. Sure, they believed the numbers, they said. But they just didn't have the time or the energy to speak out about them.

I called gynecologists around the country and asked them. Absolutely, they knew, but again, they were weary and felt helpless to succeed at anything beyond "damage control" (code words for pleading with kids to use condoms).

I called high school counselors. Did they know about this epidemic? No, they said, but they believed the numbers. "Life for many of these kids just feels out of control," many of them lamented.

So I wrote this book to bring to parents and educators the information we must have to help our own kids negotiate a very toxic sexual culture. When the first edition of this book was printed in 2002, 15.3 million Americans contracted a sexually transmitted disease each year, and two-thirds of those infections occurred in teens. We weren't immunizing young girls against HPV, and many in the general public had never heard of human papilloma virus or the vaccine for cervical cancer. Since 2002, the number of cases of new sexually transmitted diseases has jumped by *four million*—and more than half (approximately 10 million) of these infections occur in teens. In 2006 the pharmaceutical company Merck introduced a vaccine against HPV, and in short order, pediatricians across the country began immunizing girls as young as nine against this sexually transmitted disease. HPV became a household word and even kids have learned that cervical cancer is caused not by a "common" virus, but by a sexually transmitted one.

What you will read is meant to sober you and to help us as parents understand that today's sexual culture is not that of the 1970s or even the 1980s. The sexual landscape is changing fast, and sexual education programs have difficulty keeping up with the rate of infections. These infections are real, and they are broader, I believe, than any of us realize. Our kids are confused and they need honest answers, facts, and help. We owe this to them. We, the generation who birthed the sexual revolution and the feminist movement, owe our kids our best efforts to keep them from the harm that many of us unleashed on them.

Much of this information will frighten you, and you won't want to believe it. So don't take my word for it—look up the data referenced in the notes section. We are not to live fearfully, but wisely, with our eyes open and our ears ready to listen and our opinions ready to be heard. This epidemic can be reversed. It *will be* reversed because our kids get what's going on and they are backing away from sex. In 1991, 54 percent of kids were sexually active before high school graduation. That number has now dropped to 46 percent. Why? Because kids know that trouble is all around them. They realize (while we adults don't) that the sexual climate is very dangerous, and they are opting to postpone sex until they are older. Good for them.

We must educate ourselves so we can help them. Helping kids avoid sex when they are young is no longer a moral or religious issue; it is a medical one. If I didn't believe that we can be effective in helping our kids delay their sexual debut, I would stay silent. But we can help. You can help. Who you are and what you say to the teen in your life can save his life.

This book is for you. Take what you learn and change the life of one teen you know. Here are seven crucial ways to protect your kids from the deadly epidemic that has claimed far too many young lives already.

1. Know the data

Teens today face greater threats than we did, with the twin (and related) epidemics of sexually transmitted infections and depression. Know the facts to prevent your teen from becoming a victim.

2. Get to know your teen's friends

The best way to find out what your teen is involved in is to ask what his friends are up to. You can bet that whatever your kids' friends are doing, your own children are doing as well.

3. Don't just talk—listen

If you really want to get closer to your kids and get them to open up, just gently ask questions and then listen without responding or interrupting. You must wait (sometimes days) to give your opinion—if you want it to make an impression on your teen.

4. Engage, don't bail

Teens need—and want—parental involvement more than even toddlers do, even though they'll likely deny it. (An angry 16-year-old with a set of car keys is far more dangerous to himself than a 2-year-old running toward the street.) Stay connected and stay present.

5. Persevere and never take kids personally

Always remember that your job is to raise healthy adults, and screaming 13-year-olds aren't there yet. Never take juvenile hissy fits personally. Even if it seems you're not making progress, keep at it. Persistent parenting pays off in the long run.

6. Stick to your instincts

Most parents don't like skimpy clothing, vile music, or inappropriate TV shows, but they let it go because if other parents allow these things, they should too, right? Wrong. Healthy parental protection actually makes teens more secure and builds higher self-esteem. Adults' instincts are more mature than teens' instincts. Seventeen-year-olds don't have full cognitive development. She may not understand why she shouldn't wear a tiny top that leaves nothing to the imagination, but you do. If you tell her that you care about how she presents herself, she'll know how much you love her, and her self-esteem will grow.

7. Let your kids know that you are not the enemy

Often parents and kids fall into the trap of thinking that they're on opposing teams. You're not. In the great culture war for our kids, you're on the same team. The opposing team is not you and your spouse—it's the toxic popular culture that markets sex to make money off kids. That culture doesn't care about your kids' safety, health, or future. You do.

Preface

I am young for a physician. I have been seeing patients for only 20 years now. But the changes I have witnessed among the illnesses in our kids have rattled me to the core.

During my pediatric training in a large inner-city hospital, I cared for multitudes of kids with countless problems. Many of their problems centered around sex—pregnancy, STDs, and sexual abuse. It was disturbing but I kept thinking that life would be better, cleaner, less complicated once I went into a suburban private practice caring for middle-income and higher-income kids. In 1987 I left the inner city and entered private practice, and over the next several years I took care of red-faced babies who nursed beautifully. I liked leaving behind the mess.

And it seemed that for 5 years or so, the bulk of the mess did stay away. But then something happened. It came to my office, into my patients, into the schools that my patients attended. Like tiny explosions erupting around our small town, abnormal Pap smears started showing up, pelvic inflammatory diseases, herpes, and HPV came into my exam rooms like rude invaders. They didn't belong in my patients. My patients were teenagers. They weren't high risk. Most didn't have drug problems. What in the world was happening?

When I went to medical conferences around the country I asked my colleagues what they were seeing. They told me the same frightening story—STDs, risky behaviors, and in younger and younger kids. Not just in the tough crowds—in all types of crowds. I became particularly distressed talking to my gynecologist friends. They saw the messes too. They felt like they were fighting an uphill battle that couldn't be won. As they shrugged their shoulders in frustration, I began to see my patients' teachers doing the same thing. "We know our kids are having sex all the time. And we know they may get sick, but what can we do?" I heard this repeatedly from both teachers and physicians.

As my own kids have grown, I've become increasingly troubled by the advertising, the movies, and the magazines targeting our kids. Like so many other parents, I have been dragged into Abercrombie & Fitch and the video rental store, and have shaken my head "no" until it felt like it would fall off. Maybe these bother me more than most parents. Because in the morning, I drive to my office, go behind a closed examining room door, and clean up another mess. Like HPV in a 15-year-old or herpes in a high school senior.

My hope is that, as you read about my patients and you see the overwhelming data about the epidemic of STDs, you will become uncomfortable too.

My goal is not just to shock or upset you. I also want to give you tremendous encouragement. You are the answer to the epidemic surrounding all of our kids.

Acknowledgments

This work is not mine, it belongs to many who have labored hours to help produce it and endeavor to make life richer for millions of our kids.

Special thanks to Anne Mann and Sally Miller. Your belief in me and hard work for me has kept me writing; you are great friends.

To Marty Nolting, my terrific typist, thank you for your patience and your excellent work.

To Karen Anderson, thank you for your inspiration and enthusiasm.

To Mike Ward, my boss and friend at LifeLine Press, thank you for your encouragement.

To my fabulous editors, Ernie Tremblay and Molly Mullen. Without your cumulative expertise, this book might have fallen on its head. Also, thanks to Deb Gordon.

To Marji Ross at Regnery, thank you for believing in this message and giving me the opportunity to get it out.

Thanks to Tom Fitch for his expertise on condoms.

And to my mentor, Joe McIlhaney. Thank you for leadership and dedication to teens. You are my hero.

PART I

The Epidemic Is Here

ONE

■ Every year, approximately 8 million teens and young adults contract an STD. This works out to 21,000 each day.

Lori, Alex, Holly

CHANCES ARE YOU DON'T REALIZE IT, but right now, at this very minute, there is an epidemic racing through the lives of our teenagers. This epidemic literally threatens their very lives. I am a pediatrician. I see and treat these youngsters every day. I'd like you to meet some of my patients.

LORI'S STORY

As I swept the gray drapery surrounding Lori's emergency room bed behind me, I was startled by the intensity of pain I saw on her young face. Her mother said she was having abdominal discomfort, but clearly either she understated the situation or something had happened on the car ride over. This was one sick kid.

I glanced at the cardiorespiratory monitor above her head and noted that her heart was racing dangerously fast. Her breathing was labored and her blood pressure was beginning to drop. If we didn't act quickly, I realized that Lori would go into shock and die. But what was wrong? The ER physician thought she had acute appendicitis. "High fever, right-lower-quadrant pain, otherwise healthy fourteen-year-old girl—I'll bet she may have ruptured." He reassured me that the surgeon was on his way in for an emergency appendectomy.

While intravenous fluids rushed into her small veins and antibiotics were pushed into the plastic tubing by the nurse, I laid my stethoscope on her chest. Her heart was racing too fast and I didn't like her breathing pattern. I gently placed my hands on her abdomen and pressed—it felt like a piece of oak floorboard. Stiff. I was sure she'd ruptured something inside, and we needed to act immediately.

"Where are those guys? She should have been in surgery half an hour ago!" I barked at the ER nurse. "Is anesthesia ready, do they have an operating room prepared?"

"Sorry, Dr. Meeker. We had to call in another surgeon. Dr. Townsend's in surgery right now with an auto accident case," the nurse told me.

The next ten minutes felt like two hours, but finally the other surgeon appeared and whisked Lori to the OR. As I spoke with her mother and father, trying to reassure them that she was in good hands, I worried. I knew that once an abscess ruptures in the abdomen, time is of the essence.

So I changed the subject while the surgeon worked. That's all I could offer. We talked about her last basketball game, when her team played my daughter's and beat them. We all smiled at the thought of the kids playing basketball, and I felt a warmth then that I knew they didn't feel. My daughter was home in bed; theirs was struggling for her life on a steel table upstairs.

When the surgeon came out of the operating room he motioned to speak to me privately. That unnerved me, as it did her parents.

"How'd it go?" I queried.

"She's in serious danger. I have to be honest. She didn't have appendicitis." He said firmly.

"When I opened her, she had an abdomen full of pus. She had a tubo-ovarian abscess which had ruptured. I had to take her right ovary and her left one doesn't look so hot. Frankly, she'll be lucky if she pulls through," he told me.

What his findings told me was that Lori had pelvic inflammatory disease, caused by either chlamydia or gonorrhea. The infection began in her cervix and climbed to her uterus, then through her fallopian tubes and out to her ovaries. It formed an abscess on her right ovary that had ruptured, spilling the infection into her abdominal cavity. This type of infection is always life-threatening. How had she gotten the infection in the first place? Whether she had had sex once, twice, five times—it didn't matter.

When I told her parents they were shocked and frightened. Her father's instinct was to blame her boyfriend. After all, he said, he was 16 and should have known better than to harm his young daughter. Then he became angry with me, the surgeon, himself, then Lori. Then he just broke down and sobbed.

Two days passed and Lori finally turned the corner. Her heart rate returned to normal, her blood pressure rebounded, and the antibiotics we pumped into her veins seemed to be winning the battle against chlamydia. She didn't have gonorrhea, as it turned out, and this was good. Chlamydia is stubborn enough.

After a week, Lori went home from the hospital. She would live with the scar tissue surrounding her one remaining ovary and fallopian tubes for the rest of her life. It is highly unlikely that she will ever bear a child.

ALEX'S STORY

"Oh, no! Dr. Meeker, *you* can't see me. Where's the *other* Dr. Meeker? I'm supposed to see him, not you!"

"Sorry, Alex. You get me today. My husband's busy with other patients. Do you want to wait until the end of the day? He may be able to see you then."

"No. I need help, like, now. This pain is killing me."

"Okay, Alex. Why don't you tell me what's going on? Where is the pain, and when did it start?"

" I don't know what happened," said Alex. "I woke up yesterday and started feeling kinda sick. Then I felt achy all over. When I woke up today I had bumps all over my...my...private areas." He winced as he spoke and grabbed his thighs, pounding them. "I don't know what's going on. Do you think I've got cancer or something? I mean, this is bad."

"Well, let me take a look," I said. "I don't think you're going to die, and I don't think you've got cancer, but let's figure out what's going on."

Alex undressed and I indeed saw three or four blistered vesicles on his scrotum and penis. They looked like chickenpox and his genitalia were red and inflamed. I knew the signs. Alex had genital herpes.

After I finished examining him, I told Alex what he had. I told him that I could give him strong pain medication and medication to help keep the herpes under control, but that antibiotics wouldn't kill it because it was a virus. When he realized what I was saying, he sank in his chair.

Alex came back again and again. Usually he saw my husband, and I learned from him that after about five days, the herpes receded into his nervous system, as herpes typically does. My husband contacted Alex's three girlfriends and told them that they too needed to be on the lookout for genital herpes. One of them was 13 years old.

The next time I saw Alex was a year later. He was 18. He came in because he had a sore throat and, like the last time, saw me as a last resort. He was embarrassed. I could see it in the way that he hesitated to make eye contact with me. Whenever I looked at his eyes, they darted toward the floor.

As I peered down his throat, I tried to make light conversation, pretending I'd forgotten all about our last visit. But something about his inflections, his body language, and his facial expressions led me to believe that he was more than just embarrassed. After I gave him a diagnosis for his illness that day, I asked him if he was okay.

He sat silent for a few moments then broke into tears. As he cried, his whole body shook. When he quieted, I asked him how long he'd been struggling with such sadness. He told me that it started "that day." Another outbreak.

I learned more: "Something's wrong with me," he said. "I wake up in the morning and feel like someone's kicked me in the stomach. I don't care much about playing soccer anymore. My folks are on my case. We fight a lot, then I leave the house and just try to stay away."

Sleeping was an issue, too. "Once I get to sleep I don't stay there. I wake up and can't get back to sleep," Alex confessed. "By the morning I'm so tired I can barely get to school." On dating: "I don't want to date or anything. I mean, I do, but I don't. Get it? I just feel sorta messed up. I mean, I've got this DISEASE. It's scary. I don't want to have to tell a girl. If we start dating and then start having sex, what if . . . what if she finds out? I mean, she'll think I'm dirty. I guess that's it. I just feel dirty."

"Have you ever thought of killing yourself?" I asked him quietly.

He stared at me and paused before he answered. " I got some pills from my mom's bathroom and started to take some . . . . I chickened out, though," he said.

"When was that?"

"Coupla weeks ago."

HOLLY'S STORY

When I answered my page, I was startled to hear Marion's curt tone on the other end of the phone. Marion is the mother of my long-time patient Holly, and she was half angry, half upset. I had known her for years and had never heard her sound this way.

"Meg," she started, "I know you haven't seen Holly in two years and I know that you think she needs an internist now because she's gotten older. But you need to see her as soon as possible."

"What's up?" I asked.

"Holly came home from college two weeks ago and saw the gynecologist you suggested. He's scared the daylights out of both of us— he says she needs surgery. As if that weren't enough, the reason she's having problems is because of HPV. The worst part, he told me over the phone, is that she's probably had numerous infections with it over the years. Meg, she's only nineteen years old, and she could have cancer! Nobody told her this could happen. Nobody told *me*." I could hear Marion begin to cry.

"I'll see you both on Wednesday, end of the day," I said.

Marion and Holly were in the exam room right on time. I felt guilty and sad. I had known that Holly started having sex when she was 17, a junior in high school. I had told her the dangers and recommended that she tell her mother. I didn't think that this would be difficult because she and her mother were very close. She agreed, and said that she'd think about it.

Holly told me then that college and a career were very important to her, and that she certainly was going to do everything in her power to avoid getting pregnant. On at least two previous visits, Holly and I had thoroughly discussed the importance of postponing sex as long as she could. But then Holly didn't come back for office visits.

That Wednesday, we pieced together what had transpired in her life since she went away to college and moved out of my care. She decided that she really didn't want to postpone sex. She had a steady boyfriend at 17 and had felt that she was mature enough to have a sexual relationship. She got on oral contraceptives, and they had fairly regular sex for about a year. Then another "serious" boyfriend came along, and they had a sexual relationship for about six months. "Any others?" I queried.

"Well, since it's out in the open. Yeah. Two. They weren't a big deal, though. Just had sex a coupla times with each." she admitted. "After I started, I thought it was fine to just keep going."

As Holly spoke, Marion sat beside her silent.

"What did Dr. Reynolds tell you?" I asked.

"I went to see him while I was home on spring break. He did an exam and asked me a bunch of questions. About a week after I got back to school, his nurse called to say that my Pap smear was abnormal, that he wanted to see me back in his office as soon as possible.

"I was too chicken to tell Mom or anybody else. When I got there, he told me that my cervix showed signs of cancer and that I needed a LEEP procedure. I still don't get what that is. Anyway, I asked him how in the world all this happened to me. He said that I had HPV—probably several different strains of the virus—and I guess I still don't really know what that is either. No one talked about it at school that I can remember."

Holly's mom was quiet but tense, with a mixture of anger and fear. "Meg," she said, "walk us through this. What is this procedure?"

"Well, the LEEP is a fairly simple procedure done by gynecologists. LEEP stands for 'loop electrosurgical excision procedure.' Holly will go to the outpatient surgery department of the hospital and Dr. Reynolds will meet you there. He may give her a local anesthetic beforehand. Then he'll take a laser instrument and remove part of her cervix. He does this to make sure that any precancerous cells are removed so that they won't turn into more dangerous ones. Does this make sense?" I asked, to make sure that they were following everything I was telling them.

"How much will he remove?" Marion asked.

"That depends. Every woman's cervix is shaped differently and he could remove a small portion or quite a large piece, depending upon how large an area is involved."

"Will this hurt a lot?" Holly asked nervously.

"It will be uncomfortable and you'll have some cramps. You'll be able to go home shortly after it's finished," I said, trying to sound as reassuring as I knew how.

"What about children?" Marion asked.

"I'm not a gynecologist, but I will tell you that she'll be at a much higher risk for complications during her pregnancy, particularly if Dr. Reynolds has to remove a lot of tissue. The cervix helps the baby stay within the uterus during pregnancy. If he has to remove a large portion of it, she might have trouble holding her pregnancy," I said.

"But let's take one step at a time," I said. "Let Dr. Reynolds get rid of the precancerous cells. If Holly doesn't have this procedure done, untreated cervical cancer is nothing to fool around with. It is life-threatening."

"Cancer, from sex," Marion said, to nobody in particular. "She's only a freshman in college." Marion's disbelief and sadness were obvious.

Four days after our conversation, Marion held Holly's hand while Dr. Reynolds burned a piece about the size of a thick quarter out of Holly's cervix. That fall she went back to college to finish her studies in biochemical engineering. She will, I learned, have trouble bearing children, and it's likely she'll go into premature labor when she does become pregnant. "But," as Dr. Reynolds said, "it sure beats aggressive cervical cancer."

As of this writing, a year and half later, I learned from Marion that Holly's recent Pap smear results were again abnormal.

Two

■ Nearly one out of four sexually active teens is living with a sexually transmitted disease at this moment.

The Epidemic Is Real

THIS BOOK ISN'T JUST ABOUT LORI, Alex, and Holly. It is about an epidemic of sexually transmitted diseases that is invading the lives of all of our teens. It is about our future and the future of our country. It is about the suffering (both physical and emotional) occurring in the kids we love so much today, and the suffering that will occur five, 10, even 20 years from now. It's about how this epidemic will affect our children's ability to have their own, and even whether those children—our grandchildren—will live long, healthy lives or die prematurely.

Consider that this year alone, 19 million Americans will contract a new sexually transmitted disease. More to the point, 2 million to 4 million of those infected will be teenagers. Some will be infected with not just one, but two or three diseases. Overall, 25% of teens— *one out of every four adolescents*—who are sexually active will contract a sexually transmitted disease (STD) today. Even more outrageous is the fact that although teenagers make up just 10% of the population, they incur 25% of these diseases.

Every day, 21,000 teens will become infected with a new STD.[1] In fact, a British study found that almost half of all girls are likely to become infected with an STD *during their very first sexual experience.*[2] We have a serious problem on our hands.

While the statistics may shock you, they've become a part of daily life for me. Every day, one-third of the sexually active teenage patients I see have a sexually transmitted disease. Yes, I said one-third. It might be herpes, or human papilloma virus (HPV), or chlamydia. Every once in a while one turns up with gonorrhea or syphilis. More rarely, I have to tell a kid still wearing braces he has HIV, the virus that causes AIDS.

I and hundreds of doctors like me are on the front lines of this epidemic. We see precancerous conditions in girls as young as 14, infertility in girls barely old enough to get pregnant, babies infected with STDs their mothers didn't know they had, and infants born with herpes-caused encephalitis infections, which cause massive brain swelling. We see our children dying from HIV or cancer caused by HPV—dying before they've barely had a chance to live.

Public health officials call this explosion of STDs among our children a "hidden epidemic."[3] From where I sit, as a practicing adolescent doctor, I couldn't agree more.

This is an epidemic, for sure, but it is a silent epidemic. For this epidemic, there is no public outrage, no television news magazine exposé, no based-on-a-true-story movie about crusading advocates fighting this scourge, no Congressional hearings, and no Race for the Cure. And yet this epidemic is just as serious as any health emergency you can think of. It threatens the very lives of our children and the future health of our country.

It's time this epidemic comes out from the shadows. Only then, when we've begun to understand the magnitude, to comprehend the scope, to shine the light of knowledge and understanding on this terrifying scourge, can we begin talking about solutions.

And the scope is immense. Trying to wrap your mind around it is like trying to comprehend distance in light-years. Consider:

- This year, 8 to 10 million teens will contract an STD.[4]
- Nearly one out of four sexually active teens is living with a sexually transmitted disease at this moment.
- Nearly 50% of African-American teenagers have genital herpes.[5]
- Although teenagers make up just 10% of the population, they acquire between 20 and 25% of all STDs.[6]
- Herpes (specifically, herpes simplex virus type 2) has skyrocketed 500% in the past 20 years among white American teenagers.[7]
- One in five children over age 12 tests positive for herpes type 2.[8]
- Nearly one out of ten teenage girls has chlamydia, and half of all new chlamydia cases are diagnosed in girls 15 to 19 years old.[9]
- STDs accounted for 87% of all cases reported of the top-ten most frequently reported diseases in the United States in 1995.[10]

Even more terrifying is that these numbers are only guesstimates. Because most STDs have no symptoms, experts can only estimate the scope of the epidemic. The actual figures, some say, are many times higher. In February 2002, an editorial in the esteemed *Journal of the American Medical Association* reported that the number of people with asymptomatic STDs (those that have no outward signs, like lesions or warts) probably *exceeds* those whose diseases have been diagnosed.[11]

Here's another way to look at it: Picture a football stadium filled with teenagers. Start counting. One in five cheering kids has herpes.

One in four has some type of STD and one in ten has chlamydia. If we pulled all the healthy kids out of there, leaving just those teens infected with an STD, the stadium would still be nearly full.

THE EPIDEMIC DEFINED

An epidemic occurs when, in a particular community, there is an extensive and growing prevalence of a disease that attacks many people simultaneously.

Using that definition, there is no question that our teenagers are experiencing an epidemic of sexually transmitted diseases.

Epidemic is also defined as a disease that does not naturally exist within a certain place. When it comes to STDs, that place is our kids' bodies. Our teens have naturally occurring yeast and bacteria in their bodies that act to enhance their health, aiding in digestion and helping maintain healthy homeostasis. But STDs don't belong in children's bodies. They are foreign invaders. They infect healthy organs and tissues in the reproductive tracts, the bloodstreams, and the mouths of our children.

Furthermore, the STD epidemic is not a single epidemic. The Centers for Disease Control and Prevention (CDC) consider it a *multiple* epidemic of at least 25 diseases—nearly 50 if you count the various strains of virus groups. The most common STDs are HPV, herpes, chlamydia, hepatitis B, gonorrhea, syphilis, HIV/AIDS, trichomoniasis, and chancroid. And there are a host of others that threaten our kids, most with only clinical names that sound as foreign as another universe. Consider some of them: *Mycoplasma hominis*; *Ureaplasma urealyticum*; bacterial vaginosis; granuloma inguinale; shigellosis; *Campylobacter*; hepatitis A, C, and D; cytomegalovirus; genital molluscum contagiosum; human T-cell lymphotrophic virus types 1 and 2; amebiasis; *Giardia*; and *Candida albicans*.

All of these wreak havoc on young bodies in different ways; some work quickly, some take their toll slowly.

It's so hard to grasp the vastness of these infections. Just picture flying 10,000 feet above Yellowstone National Park, looking out the window, and seeing thousands of small fires. Some are blazing and spreading, others crackle and smolder, and still others just spit out some smoke and a few sparks. Although they all have varying degrees of seriousness, when you're flying at 10,000 feet, all those flames merge and the entire park appears engulfed in fire. That's what's happening to the population of our kids.

LIFELONG, LIFE-THREATENING

In the 1960s, a simple shot of penicillin could cure the two known STDs: syphilis and gonorrhea. Today, there are no simple cures and *in many cases there are no cures at all.*

Take herpes. Currently, more than 45 million Americans are infected with the herpes simplex type 2 virus because there is no way to cure it. A 1997 study published in *The New England Journal of Medicine* sent shock waves through the medical community when its authors reported that 20% of those 12 and older tested positive for this strain of herpes.[12] Initially, I, like many physicians and parents I speak to, assumed the researchers were testing people in STD clinics. So of course the numbers would be high; these people are going to the clinic because they think they have an STD. But that was not the case. The researchers tested people in the general population, *not groups of people with high-risk behavior.* When I tell audiences about this, many don't believe me. I had to read the article twice to believe it myself.

Overall, teenagers today are five times more likely to have herpes than they were in the 1970s.[13]

This should terrify you as much as it does me, since herpes spreads *only* through sexual contact, and can remain hidden with no symptoms for months or years. Herpes is a lifelong disease that can resurface again and again, causing bouts of painful genital ulcers, disrupting lives, putting barriers between its victim and his or her partner, providing a constant reminder of mistakes made 10, 20, 30 years ago. Not something you want your teenager to live with.

Or consider HPV, one of the most prevalent sexually transmitted diseases in this country. HPV is the infection most responsible for my personal crusade to help teenagers avoid sex. It has the dubious distinction of being one of the few causes of cancer we know about, and is responsible for 99.7% of cervical cancer cases and the deaths of nearly 5000 women each year.[14]

Men aren't safe from HPV's devastating effects either. The virus is linked to penile and anal cancer, and troubling new research suggests it may also play a role in some head and neck cancers.[15] Although vaccines are being researched, nothing is available today to the general public. Likewise, there is no medication, no treatment that will eliminate the virus. Just careful watching for the first precancerous cells to appear. Even worse: *Most victims have no symptoms* (just 1% develop genital warts). Having this virus without knowing it is like living with a ticking time bomb.

Then there's HIV, the virus that causes AIDS. You've no doubt heard of the nearly miraculous new drugs for HIV, medications that significantly improve the quality and duration of life for those infected with the virus. Those medications, however, haven't changed the ultimate truth about AIDS: It is fatal.

And although the majority of HIV cases still occur between men having sex with men, the number of HIV-infected women is rising rapidly. In 2000, nearly half (45%) of all AIDS cases among 13- to 24-year-old women were acquired through heterosexual sex.[16] Here's an even more frightening number: *More than half (61%)* of young people between 13 and 19 who were infected with HIV that year were women.[17] *More young women than young men are getting HIV.* Again, the disproportion exists even within HIV: Half of all new infections are in our youth![18]

Even if your child is "lucky" enough to catch a "curable" STD, such as chlamydia or gonorrhea, there's no guarantee that we, her health care providers, will catch and cure it before it causes significant damage. In young girls, for instance, the bacteria that cause these infections can "escape" from the cervical area (where we can get a culture and identify it) into the uterus and up through the fallopian tubes, causing a secondary infection called pelvic inflammatory disease (PID). As it races through their bodies, PID leaves girls' fallopian tubes and ovaries severely scarred and permanently damaged, perhaps rendering these girls infertile, or subject to a potentially fatal tubal pregnancy. We've seen PID rates skyrocket in the past 15 years. Today, almost a quarter of a million teenagers are diagnosed with PID every year, as a direct result of the spread of STDs— and chlamydia and gonorrhea in particular.[19]

The spread of gonorrhea, one of the oldest STDs, was coming down in numbers until the late 1990s, when the rate of infection began inching up again. If you think this STD isn't worth worrying about because a quick dose of antibiotics can cure it, think again. Today, public health officials are alarmed by rising numbers of antibiotic-resistant strains of gonorrhea. And because gonorrhea, like chlamydia, rarely announces its presence with symptoms, teenagers infected with it are at risk for a host of more serious complications, including PID.

STDS DON'T DISCRIMINATE

The next time you're at the mall, take a moment to observe that pack of teens you're likely to see roaming the storefronts. Chances are good you'll spot a bright young girl sporting a stomach-baring tank top. Even as she window-shops at American Eagle Outfitters, there's a one in four likelihood that a virus is working its way up through her reproductive tract, changing the cells in her cervix so that in a few months, maybe in a few years, she'll find she has a precancerous condition requiring surgery. You may spot a boy in low-rider jeans and a backwards-turned baseball cap. Chances are one in twenty that he's got a sore on his penis he's too embarrassed to ask anyone about. Even if he did get up the courage to ask, he's not sure *whom* to confide in. And that group of ten girls moving together like a school of brightly colored tropical fish? At least one has a bacterial infection she doesn't know about, an infection that will leave her infertile.

We're not talking about troubled teens: We're talking about *all* teens—yours and mine. The teens who belong to the church youth group, work at the local gas station, or hand you ice cream across the counter. They have personalities and faces. Look at their faces and see who you think might be infected. If you look at more than five, chances are you'll see at least one infected with a horrible disease.

Black, white, Asian, Hispanic. Rich kids or poor. Straight-A students or dropouts. It doesn't matter. Sexually transmitted viruses, bacteria, and parasites don't discriminate. They attack all sexually active teens. Consider just one example:

An astonishing 15 to 20% of all young men will be infected with the herpes virus by the time they reach adulthood.[20]

LIKE A MATCH TO GASOLINE

The reasons for the current epidemic among our children are clear. I'll outline just a few of them here; later in the book, I'll go into much more detail.

Birth control and condoms. Public health officials and doctors have been fighting teen pregnancy for decades now with two heavy-duty weapons: oral contraceptives and condoms. The overwhelming goal that we've dealt with has been to reduce teen pregnancy. Congratulations: Teen pregnancy dipped in the late 1990s, and now every year, about 1 million teen girls get pregnant.

I myself worked for nearly a decade prescribing birth control to teens. I believed that oral contraception was the most powerful weapon I had to help teens avoid life-altering dilemmas that can and do cause irreversible physical and psychological harm. But I realize now that what we've been doing has been akin to rearranging the deck chairs on the Titanic. We now face a gargantuan consequence of that sexual freedom: At the same time teen pregnancies declined, the STD epidemic shot through the roof. The sexual freedom that birth control allows teens has done a good deal to promote the rise in disease.

Condoms are no answer either. As you'll see in Chapter 7, condoms do little to prevent many viral infections spread by skin-to-skin contact, especially HPV and herpes. We've talked for decades about "safe sex," and while condoms are somewhat effective at birth control, when it comes to STDs, the best they can do is reduce the risk of infection. And the risk of reduction, as you'll see, is far too inadequate and in some cases nonexistent.

What they don't know *can* hurt them. If you figured the sex education classes your teenager takes in middle and high school would include information about STDs, think again. One study found that most teens fail a simple test on their knowledge of STDs. When researchers gave 66 young adults (13 to 24 years old) attending a health fair a 13-question exam, most came up with only six correct answers.[21] Some of the questions stumped nearly everyone.

Four out of five, for example, didn't know that most people who get an STD never develop symptoms.[22]

They're starting too young. Half of all students in ninth through twelfth grade have had sexual intercourse. This is particularly dangerous, since studies show that the earlier a teen begins having sex, the more partners he or she will have. In fact, of those having sex, between 12 and 20% have had *four or more sexual partners* in their young lives.[23] The more partners, the more exposure to infection. The 17-year-old who's had six sexual partners (all of whom have had six sexual partners, and so on and so on) may have been exposed to the diseases of 63 people.

I cannot stress this enough:

The longer a teen can wait to begin sexual activity, the less likely it is that he or she will contract a sexually transmitted disease.

They're confused about what "sex" means. Millions of American teenagers have seen infamous sex scandals unfold on the six-o'clock news, codes of acceptable language disappear from television and popular music, and an inescapable deluge of sexual images floods movies, electronic games, magazines, and comic books. Sexual pictures, stories, and advertising copy pop up on their computer screens while they're doing their homework. No wonder the very definition of sex seems unclear to our kids.

Out of the thousands of teens I've counseled, most reason they can safely engage in oral sex and "outercourse" (in which they mutually masturbate with their clothes off). To them, these activities are acceptable recreation, not "real" sex. Since semen doesn't enter the vagina, kids think they're playing it safe, while still maintaining their virginity and staying disease-free. So today they're having oral sex in the back of school buses and in dark movie theaters. (Ask any middle school teacher.)

And oral sex is becoming a fad with kids. Very recent studies show that even oral herpes has shifted from causing 25% of genital herpes infections to 75% of them.[24] How? Through oral sex. Here's another oral sex statistic if you want one: An online sex survey done by *Twist* magazine found that out of 10,000 girls who responded, over half (5,700) were under 14. Amazingly, 25% of girls who said they were virgins responded that they engaged in oral sex.[25]

Unfortunately, just because they're avoiding penetration doesn't mean they're avoiding disease. Many of these infections can spread simply from any sexual contact—mouth to penis, semen to skin—without intercourse.

Teens are also having group sex, and moving from one relationship to another, often within weeks or even days. Some engage in such behavior for the thrill or because they're bored. Others do it to be popular with their peer group. If you think your kid could never do such things, think again. Peer pressure is subtle, pervasive, and powerful. For the sake of your kids, you cannot afford to be naïve. You need to know exactly what your teen is up to sexually. Your child's life depends upon it.

Teenage anatomy and health. There are differences in a teenage girl's anatomy that make her far more vulnerable to infection than an adult woman is. For instance, the cells covering a teenage girl's cervix are physiologically different from the cells lining a 25- or 30-year-old woman's cervix, and are therefore far more susceptible to infections.

Treating sexually active teens is also more difficult because many parents stop taking their children to pediatricians for regular checkups and immunizations after age 10 or 12. Yet it is precisely during those adolescent years that health needs climb and teenagers desperately need someone to talk to. I've found that most of the kids who are reluctant to tell their parents they're sexually active are relieved to finally tell someone else—their doctor, for instance. So even if your teenager is healthy and you're certain he's not sexually active, please, take him to see a family physician at least once a year.

Because teens often have questions about psychological issues, their own development, or sex, make sure you choose a doctor who knows how to talk to teenagers, and is willing to give these kids all the time they need to discuss whatever's on their minds. I always schedule my teenage patients for 45-minute visits (instead of the 15-minute visits younger children get) because I know we'll do so much talking.

Allyson's Story

Allyson, a 14-year-old patient of mine, is a perfect example of what I see happening with teens. I'd been seeing her for yearly medical checkups since she was 3 years old. But when she turned 11, her mother stopped bringing her in. Shortly after her 14th birthday, however, Allie returned to my office complaining that she "just wasn't feeling good." Her mother said she'd become irritable, was difficult to be around, and was beginning to run with "the wrong crowd." While her behavior could have been passed off as that of a "normal teen" experiencing some adjustment difficulties, Allyson's mother was finely tuned in to her daughter's moods and knew something was wrong.

I immediately noticed the change in Allyson's physical appearance from the last time I'd seen her. She'd developed quickly, and appeared much older than 14. She wore tight, low-slung pants and a short-cropped shirt that flaunted her well-developed chest. Several holes pierced her earlobes, which peeked out from beneath her long, silky, auburn hair.

After Allyson's mother described her concerns, I asked her to leave, then turned to Allyson. "What do you think about what your mother just told me?" I asked.

Allyson agreed with her mother's descriptions. She said she often felt sad and angry, yet didn't have a clue what was wrong with her. "And I fight and yell a lot," she said, "without understanding why."

As she talked, I could see how relieved she felt to finally let out her concerns. Eventually, after much probing and backtracking, Ally revealed that much of her irritability had begun about six months before. She cried as she described the event that, we concluded, had turned her life upside down.

She'd heard some kids were going to have a "rainbow party," but had no idea what that meant. Still, she thought it might be fun, and arranged to attend with a friend. After she arrived, several girls (all in the eighth grade) were given different shades of lipstick and told to perform oral sex on different boys to give them "rainbows." Once she realized what was happening, Allyson was too stunned and frightened to do anything. When a girl gave her some lipstick, she refused at first but, with repeated pressure, finally gave in. "It was one of the grossest things I've ever done," she told me, crying. Afterward, she said, "I just wanted to hide and die. I felt like vomiting."

When it was over, she couldn't even look at the boy on whom she'd performed oral sex. Over the next several weeks and months, her crying spells and bouts with self-disgust felt overwhelming. Her self-esteem plummeted, and her angry eruptions at her mother, who was the person closest to her in the whole world, precipitated a breakdown in their relationship. She began dressing in sexually explicit ways, garnering attention from boys while at the same time hating their attention. Within a few months, she began having intercourse with boys. This was the point Allyson had reached when her mother brought her in to see me.

I checked Allyson for sexually transmitted diseases and, fortunately, didn't find any. I also performed a Pap smear, checking for any precancerous changes in her cervix that could have been caused by HPV. Again she was fortunate—I didn't see anything suspicious. However, I knew from long experience as a physician that she was quite likely to go on and become even more sexually active. And it was equally likely that most of the other girls—and boys—at the party would continue to be sexually active.

I spent a long time with Allyson that day, reassuring her that her feelings of sadness and disgust were normal, healthy reactions to the trauma she had been through. She had begun to believe she was going crazy because the other kids around her seemed to believe what happened was okay.

Allyson was suffering from depression and post-traumatic stress disorder. We talked that day about depression and she agreed to get help. For the next nine months, she saw a counselor once a week. Today, she's doing well. She's more careful in choosing her friends, although she has difficulty trusting people. She no longer wears sexually explicit outfits, and she abandoned her black clothing as her depression lifted. But after two years, she still needs more time to heal.

Allyson was and is a normal, healthy, all-around great kid who happened to be in the wrong place at the wrong time. Because of that, however, I have to see her every six months to check for precancerous changes or other "hidden" STDs, and the emotional scars of her experience will remain for life.

But at least Allyson got help. I often wonder how many more Allysons are roaming our high schools, feeling depressed and crazy from one, two, or three similar sexual episodes. Because I know, based on the hundreds of teenage girls I see and talk to, that only a handful say they enjoy the experience. If it were just a matter of kids doing something they didn't like, I wouldn't care. Let them do crazy stuff if it doesn't hurt them or anyone else. But sex *does* hurt our teens, physically and emotionally, and we must care enough to get in the way.

BREAKING THE SILENCE

I've been lecturing on adolescent sexuality and high-risk behavior in teens for more than six years. Everywhere I go, I hear the same question from parents, doctors, and educators: Why didn't we know about this? Where has this data been?

It's been right in front of us. But we haven't wanted to see it. We live in a world so saturated with sexuality that we no longer know the meaning of it. Television, movies, magazines, and music tell us what we want to hear: Sex is fun, and has no attached repercussions, certainly no diseases.

Mayhem in the Media

Consider *Friends*, one of the top-rated television shows for the past several years. Here we see half a dozen young people sleeping with each other or with other people while rarely making a peep about protecting themselves from sexually transmitted diseases. Statistically speaking, at least one character in the show—Monica? Joey?—*must* have an STD, but we never hear about that. Instead, in the rarefied world of *Friends*, the only repercussions to sleeping around are pregnancy and the occasional heartbreak.

In the music media, the images are even more suggestive. Popular music blares out sexually explicit lyrics. CDs are filled with line after line of expletives and raunchy themes, such as those, for example, from the popular hip-hop rapster Ja Rule.

In one song from a current CD, "Livin' It Up," this singer calls women "bitches," sings about "s*cking d*ck," "f***ing," having phone sex, and in general treating women in abusive ways. In another song, "Always on Time," he raps about sex being a game, "smacking your *ss," and "f***ing you all wild." These are just a very few illustrations in any one track.[26]

Consider another popular artist, Lil' Kim. Her song titles alone, such as "S*ck My D*ck" and "F**k You," tell an indecent story. In addition, you may be surprised to hear the sentiments in songs such as "How Many Licks," in which she sings about "Dan," her "nigga from Down South," and how he liked her to "spank him" and have her "c*m in his mouth." The song goes on to list a number of "lovers," and depicts graphic images of oral sex, rough sex, large sex organs, and dominance.[27]

One more example: Kid Rock, another artist popular with teens, who created the song "F**k Off" in 1998. Here, the Kid has been "f***ing all your bitches," and, as he says, "don't f***ing give a goddamn." In another verse, Kid Rock says he won't leave a party until he sees "naked bitches" dancing drunk and "touchin' each other." The chorus: "F**k Off."[28]

(Author's note: I've used paraphrases and images from these songs to give you an idea of the baseness of the sentiments being communicated to our kids. It was tough enough to even type the above paragraphs, let alone read the actual lyrics. But I encourage you to do so to see firsthand the brutal sexual messages that exist here. Note, too, that these are popular artists. Incredibly, some of rapper Eminem's lyrics are even worse; he writes about raping then killing women. This is "popular" stuff with many kids across all social and economic ranges.)

And yet, while the media aggressively and persistently sells sex and sexual freedoms to us and our children, doctors like me "mop up the messes" every day in our offices.

Curriculum for the Classroom

There is another even more worrisome reason for our ignorance: a conspiracy operating behind the scenes of public school sex education. Just a handful of writers design the curriculum for these classes, affecting millions of American children with their decisions and their agenda. And I do believe they have an agenda: to maintain sexual freedoms rather than prevent disease, maximize psychological health, and ensure healthy sexuality among our teens.

Just consider the guidelines from the Sexuality Information and Education Council of the United States (SIECUS), an advocacy organization that has heavily influenced the sex education curriculum in many of our public schools. The purpose of the guidelines is to provide a framework for educators who wish to teach our children about sex. The claim is that sex education "assists children in understanding a positive view of sexuality, provides them with information and skills about taking care of their sexual health, and helps them acquire skills to make decisions now and in the future." Do the SIECUS guidelines live up to that claim? Here are a few of them. Decide for yourself.

■ **For children ages 5 to 8**
- Sexual intercourse occurs when a man and woman place the penis inside the vagina.
- Touching and rubbing one's own genitals to feel good is called masturbation.
- Boys and girls have body parts that feel good when touched.
- Some men and women are homosexual, which means that they

will be attracted to and fall in love with someone of the same gender.

■ For children ages 9 to 12

- Words related to sexuality that may be appropriate with friends may not be appropriate at school, home, or work.
- Masturbation is often the first way a person experiences sexual pleasure.
- Being sexual with another person usually involves more than sexual intercourse.
- Sexual intercourse provides pleasure.
- When a man and woman want to have vaginal intercourse without having a child, they can use contraception to prevent pregnancy.
- Homosexual love relationships can be as fulfilling as heterosexual relationships.

■ For children ages 12 to 15

- People should use contraception during vaginal intercourse unless they want to have a child.
- Masturbation, either alone or with a partner, is one way a person can enjoy and express their sexuality without risking pregnancy or an STD/HIV.
- When two people express their sexual feelings together, they usually give and receive pleasure.
- Being sexual with another person usually involves different sexual behaviors.
- People may fantasize while they are alone or with a partner.
- Having an abortion rarely interferes with a woman's ability to become pregnant or give birth in the future.

■ **For children ages 15 to 18**

- Some sexual behaviors shared by partners include kissing;
  touching; talking; caressing; massaging; sharing erotic literature
  or art; bathing or showering together; and oral, vaginal, or anal
  intercourse.
- Some people use erotic photographs, movies, or literature to
  enhance their sexual fantasies when alone or with a partner.
- Some sexual fantasies involve mysterious or forbidden things.
- Most people enjoy giving and receiving pleasure.

Once you review these statements, it seems clear that SIECUS
places sexual freedom for teens above their health. As long as the
idea of sexual freedom remains the driving force behind national sex
education, the STD epidemic will continue.

In many ways our efforts as a society and, in some instances, as parents to be open-minded and mature about our children's sexuality, to
understand their sexual freedoms, have backfired. Many parents were
taught that one cannot judge youngsters who choose early sexual
activity because to do so would violate some inalienable personal right.
Some parents and educators find themselves trapped in a no-man's-
land: believing in personal and sexual freedom, yet facing deadly diseases spawned by unrestrained and premature sexual activity.

The epidemic of STDs our children face is too serious to ignore.
The only way to stop it is to curb the conspiracy of those who urge
total sexual freedom and argue that it has no costs and causes no
harm.

How do we do this? We must stand between our kids and the
media and big businesses who aggressively sell them sex. If we fail to
teach teens to postpone sex as long as possible, the price they pay
may be their very lives.

Teaching them won't be easy. Some won't listen. Some will argue.
Some will nod their heads at everything we say, then go off and do

as they please. But with patience, honesty, and determination, we can help them understand. And we must. As parents and concerned adults who love the children in our lives, it is our responsibility to do so. The other piece of the puzzle—knowledge, based both on solid research and on real-life experience—is what I hope you will find in the chapters ahead.

THREE

■ There are approximately 30 strains of human papilloma virus, which cause genital infections; HPV causes 99.7% of all cervical cancers.

The Explosion
from Two to Twenty-five

IN 1960, PHYSICIANS CONTENDED with two major sexual diseases: gonorrhea and syphilis. We thought of them as problems limited to sailors and prostitutes. No one talked about them. If you experienced some strange symptoms in, on, or near your reproductive organs, you sheepishly headed to your doctor for an injection of penicillin, then tried to forget the experience.

As I talk to older doctors and learn about those early days of "VD," I envy the simplicity of them. Those early diseases were cured with that shot of penicillin. Once treated, they didn't linger for a lifetime, causing the long-term complications we face today, including death.

Today we're faced with the ravages of far more than those two simple STDs: we're battling scores of viruses and bacteria. With multiple strains of mutating viruses, and the emergence of some antibiotic-resistant bacteria, *the actual number of true STDs we face may be as high as 35 to 40.*

How did this happen?

As the "free-love" movement of the 1960s gained momentum and the barriers around sexual activity dissolved, doctors began seeing a slew of new viruses and bacteria.

Take chlamydia, for instance. We didn't even identify it until 1976. Today it's the most commonly transmitted bacterial STD in this country. Teenagers roll the word off their tongues as easily as we did "Woodstock."

In 1982, genital herpes was so commonplace that *Time* magazine made it the subject of one of its covers, under the headline: "VD of the Ivy League." Today, more than 40 million Americans are infected with this virus.[1] Soon after herpes pushed its way into our consciousness, HIV and AIDS came along. When I began medical school in 1980, we'd never heard of those diseases. By the time I graduated in 1984, it was being called an epidemic. Nine years later, between 1 million and 2 million Americans were infected with HIV or AIDS, over 12 million worldwide, and more than 160,000 had died in the United States alone. By 1994, AIDS had become the leading cause of death for people between the ages of 25 and 40. Currently, the virus has killed more Americans (450,000) than died throughout all of World War II.[2]

Before 1985, we rarely saw cases of human papilloma virus (HPV). Today, it is believed to be the most prevalent STD of all. Studies show that 20 million people that we know of are infected now, but 80 million Americans are believed to have been infected with genital HPV at some point in their lives.[3] In 1996, it was identified as the definitive cause of nearly all cervical cancers, a disease limited only one generation ago to women 55 and older. The infection is now prevalent in teenagers, and the highest incidence is in young women under 25.[4]

By 1990, penicillin-resistant strains of gonorrhea were present in all fifty states, and by 1992 syphilis was at a 20-year high.[5] By 1993, pelvic inflammatory disease (PID), almost always caused by gonorrhea or chlamydia, was being diagnosed in 1 million women a year. Among them were 200,000 teenagers, at least one-fourth of whom would suffer long-term damage.[6] The trend has continued. In fact, next to pregnancy, PID is now the leading cause of hospitalization for women between the ages of 15 and 55.[7]

In a mere four decades, we witnessed STDs move through our society from the promiscuous to the sophisticated to the young. And adult diseases, such as cervical cancer, PID, genital herpes, and HIV, have become diseases of children.

With the exception of the influenza pandemic in 1918-19, I can't think of another time in recent history when such a devastating plague has spread so rapidly throughout the world's population.

What is the reason for the speed and magnitude of this epidemic? Simply put, the sexual revolution. With the coming of that revolution, my own generation demanded previously unheard-of sexual freedom and promiscuity. We may have gotten what we thought we wanted, but the ride wasn't free. Countless children are now paying the price. Over half admit they've had sex with two or more partners, often concurrently. And to make things more frightening, only 35%, or one in three teens, uses condoms with any consistency.[8]

Under these conditions, of course, STDs spread like wildfire. The earlier teens become sexually active, the more likely they will be to have multiple sexual partners. If a girl starts having sex before she's 16, there's a 58% chance that she'll have more than five partners. If she starts before she's 18, she'll have a 30% chance of having more than five partners.[9] The more partners you have, the greater the likelihood of catching a disease from one of them. It's like playing Russian roulette. The more times you spin the barrel, the greater your chances of getting killed. Yet, until fairly recently, we've treated sexual diseases as if they were an acceptable cost of being a sophisticated and sexually liberated society.

What a mistake we've made.

SICK FOR LIFE

The biggest change we've seen in STDs in this century is the onslaught of viral infections. Sexually transmitted viral diseases are the most frustrating for physicians because we don't have medicines to kill the bugs. We can prescribe drugs to help control the symptoms of some viral STDs, but we can't eliminate the infections from the body. Once you catch one of these nasty infections, it could be yours for life.

If only our kids understood this. Too often, a teen won't take the threat of STDs seriously because he or she believes modern medicine can cure anything with a pill or injection. Unfortunately, this couldn't be further from the truth.

Viruses are sneaky little germs. They need host cells in order to replicate. They find those cells in the tissue and blood of human beings. When they invade, they enter some of our cells, reproduce, and eventually kill the cells. Viruses may remain in the body for weeks, months, or even years. Sometimes during this period they may produce symptoms such as warts or ulcers, but most of the time they remain hidden, without producing any symptoms.

Even when they seem dormant, however, they remain very contagious. They continue to reproduce, passing their replicants on to anyone who comes in contact with infected tissue in a process called "shedding." This occurs when a virus moves to a certain spot in the body, say vaginal tissues or the nose. The virus remains there without causing any symptoms, but it can spread to other people and cause them to be infected. If you have an infection like herpes, there is no way to know when you're shedding. You won't feel any burning or tingling, or see any changes in the surface of your skin. During this time of active contagion, the carrier—who may be any teen—may have no idea he or she is even infected.

That's one reason HIV spreads so silently. It may be a very long time before someone infected with the virus knows he has it. Even an HIV blood test can miss an infection. In fact, teens with HIV are more infectious right *before* any blood test would turn positive for HIV.[10] Thus, years may go by during which an unsuspecting carrier spreads the disease through "unprotected" sex.

Your immune system is used to fighting viruses, and sometimes it even wins, as is almost always the case with the common cold. But other viruses may stay in your body for years at a time, destroying cells and in some instances making you more vulnerable to other infections. For instance, people with herpes are more vulnerable to HIV.

What follows is a primer, so to speak. It's an in-depth rundown of the most prevalent viruses that affect our kids. I can't list all the numerous viruses here—there are too many. But I can give you the lowdown on the most gnarly ones, especially the ones I've seen and treated in my own practice. Here's a quick lesson in how these viruses react, what they do to the bodies of our teens, how they're spread, and how easily they can be transmitted.

HPV: GROUND ZERO

I recently spoke to 300 ninth-grade students at a public junior high school. We talked about sex—its risks and benefits. As I talked, I delighted in watching their reactions. One group began to giggle, becoming red-faced and embarrassed—quite a healthy response. Another group rolled their eyes and emphatically gestured to me (the outdated mother) that what I was teaching was "old news." And some were disgusted by the whole suggestion of sex. They moaned, looked away, and talked to those around them. Their responses reminded me that as sophisticated and knowledgeable as we assume our teenagers to be, at heart they're still children—confused, excited, and frightened by thoughts of sex and sexuality. All good reactions.

Then I started talking about STDs. Many had heard about chlamydia, HIV, and AIDS, but few recognized HPV. (Even many adults are unaware of this viral disease.) Some kids were astute enough to associate the virus with genital warts. "Oh, yeah, we know all about those," they declared.

"What else does HPV cause—does anyone know?" I asked. There was stony silence. Even the health education teacher was silent.

"What about cervical cancer?" I asked. "Has anyone heard of that?" "Cancer? Cancer?" I heard someone yell. "You can't get cancer from sex!" Most of the students laughed.

If only that were true.

HPV, one of the most common sexually transmitted diseases, with an estimated 5.5 million new cases a year, causes more than 99.7% of all cervical cancers.[11] "When I began practicing 18 years ago, cervical cancer was a disease of older [55- to 70-year-old] women," my colleague, Michael Aja, M.D., head of the Radiation Oncology Department at Munson Hospital in Traverse City, Michigan, told me. "Today, we commonly treat young women in their 20s with cervical cancer because they got HPV infections during their younger years." Overall, 15,700 new cases of cervical cancer appear each year, with women between the ages of 22 and 25 most likely to develop it. And every year, nearly 5,000 women die from this disease.[12]

When I began my pediatric residency in 1984, I hardly ever saw precancerous cervical changes in teenage girls. But over the past 18 years, abnormal Pap smear results have become commonplace in my practice. Remember, I'm not an internist or a gynecologist. I am a pediatrician caring for children and adolescents.

About 30 types of HPV are sexually transimtted. The virus works by infecting mucous membranes in the body (vagina, cervix, mouth), and it shows a special predilection for young girls. Their young bodies have receptive vaginal mucus that easily holds the virus, and their cervical cells are more receptive to viral infections, allowing the viruses to reproduce easily. As women age, they're better able to fight off the virus, which is why rates of HPV infection in teens can be as high as 40%, compared with less than 15% in the adult population.[13] Teenagers are also more likely to develop pre-cancerous growths as a result of HPV. These growths are more likely to develop into full-blown cancer. Why, we don't know. Researchers suspect it simply has to do with the immaturity of the teen's immune system compared with that of an adult woman. In the past ten years, HPV has spread like wildfire through our country. In 1994, there were an estimated 2.5 million infections a year. Today, that figure has doubled.[14] One study found that HPV was five times more common than all other viral STDs combined![15]

And those numbers are only guesstimates, since physicians aren't required to report HPV infections to their local health departments (unlike syphilis, gonorrhea, and AIDS). Many patients aren't routinely cultured for the virus, and, most importantly, hundreds of thousands of those infected never seek medical attention because they don't have any symptoms.

In the public at large, HPV has been found in approximately 75% of sexually active people.[16] A British study found the virus infects at least 46% of teenage girls after their *first sexual intercourse*. The mind-boggling prevalence and ease of transmission led the researchers on that study to conclude, "Perhaps cervical (HPV) infection should now be considered an inevitable consequence of sexual activity."[17]

But cervical cancer is just one danger from HPV. The virus is also linked to vulvar, vaginal, uterine, and anal cancers. Infants born to infected mothers can develop wartlike tumors on their vocal cords. Men can get penile and anal cancers from HPV.[18] And HPV doesn't stop there. A study in *The New England Journal of Medicine* found that patients with certain head and neck cancers were twice as likely to have been infected with HPV in the past. Researchers speculate that the rising incidence of oral sex—and the transmission of oral HPV—contributes to these cancers.[19]

Less serious are the genital warts that HPV can cause. They appear small and flat, and, when tucked inside a teenage girl's labia, remain out of sight and mind. While they don't hurt, they can grow quite large, taking on a "cauliflower" appearance. They can even occur around the anus. Perhaps if they were more prevalent, we'd identify more cases of HPV. But only about 1% of sexually active teens and adults who have HPV have these warts. Fortunately, the warts can be treated with a prescription medication called podophyllin. If the medicine doesn't work, the wart may have to be surgically removed. *But removing the wart does not cure the disease.*

We don't have any antiviral medications to fight HPV, as we do with herpes. It's also difficult for sexually active teens to protect themselves from HPV infections because the virus spreads from skin to skin. It can be found anywhere on the genital area, and can even be spread from hand and finger contact. So condoms aren't much help.

Since HPV can't be killed and condoms don't adequately protect against its spread, the most critical factor in preventing cervical cancer is to make sure sexually active teens have a Pap test every 12 months, which is time enough for a precancerous abnormality to develop. If dysplasia, or cervical cells that have already started changing toward cancerous cells, is found, a gynecologist may need to surgically remove the affected tissue.

As recently as 2004, HPV (or human papilloma virus) was not a household word. Three years later, it is. Even grade-schoolers recognize that it, like HIV and AIDS, is just another one of those "diseases" that has always been around but that many grown-ups don't want to talk about. Cervical cancer, HPV, vaccines—they all kind of run together; young people hear them talked about (at least during their annual school check-ups) but they feel confused and distant from the whole discussion.

To many kids in grade school and junior high, HPV joins the growing and lengthy list of infections that "other kids" get when they have sex and don't use condoms.

Dr Julie Gerberding, head of the Centers for Disease Control and Prevention, recognized the seriousness of HPV and cervical cancer and issued a report to Congress. Dr. Gerberding wanted to address ways in which educators and physicians could contain the spread of HPV infections. I was fortunate to testify at the hearing and heard physicians like myself insist before Congress that HPV wreaks havoc in the young bodies of our healthy patients. I'm certain that many of us physicians held opposing political views, but those didn't come into play. We were there because, in spite of our sociopolitical differences, we wanted less cervical cancer in our patients. We wanted to increase public awareness and support Dr. Gerberding's bold statements.

What made her report worthy of mention on prime-time news broadcasts? She said that HPV is the cause of cervical cancer. That went over easily. Then she said that HPV is transmitted through sexual activity. There was the rub. Cancer from sex?

Her recommendation? "The surest way to eliminate the risk for future genital HPV infections is to refrain from any genital contact with another individual." Stop having sex? Isn't that a moral, political, or religious dictum? How could the head of a science organization make such a statement?

The report continued: "For those who choose to be sexually active, a long-term, mutually monogamous relationship with an uninfected partner is the strategy most likely to prevent future genital HPV infections."

Let's get this right. Dr. Gerberding, recognizing the seriousness of cervical cancer, wrote a statement informing Congress that if we Americans want to avoid getting cervical cancer, we had better change our sexual behavior. What about condoms? What about our right to sexual freedom? There was no discussion of that. The reason she recommends that physicians, educators, and parents teach kids to avoid sexual activity (or genital contact) is simple. HPV spreads via skin-to-skin contact. And as condoms have a poor track record of reducing the risk of contracting HPV, she recommends sticking to one partner and staying faithful to that one partner. Abstinence or monogamy, that was it. That was the solution she issued to Congress after weighing all the complexities about HPV and its spread.

Think about the ramifications of her message. Where the teaching of condom use dominated the mantra of sex ed teachers and parents across the country for decades, Dr. Gerberding claimed that condom use wasn't effective at preventing HPV and cervical cancer.

We know that she was absolutely right. Two years later, in 2006, Merck pharmaceuticals launched Gardasil, the HPV vaccine. It quickly garnered the approval of the FDA. In short order, medical organizations like the American College of Obstetrics and Gynecology recommended that physicians and health clinics across the country begin immunizing 9- to 26-year-old girls and women. Gardasil brought HPV and discussions about cervical cancer to the kitchen table. But they remain sticky words. We approach them as grade-school children approach HIV and AIDS. Yes, cervical cancer can be uncomfortable to talk about, but the real rub comes from the realization that cervical cancer is acquired through having sex. We want to change the cancer part. Of course, we also want to stamp out the STD part, but we don't want to confront the reality that the bug is outsmarting our best efforts (to date) of prevention. The only way to keep the germs at bay is to change our sexual behavior. Ouch.

Twenty million Americans currently have HPV infections, and 5.5 million people contract new HPV infections every year.[20] Do all these infections ultimately cause cervical cancer? No. Some advance to what we call cervical dysplasias and are caught before full-blown cancer occurs. There are different stages of cervical dysplasia. Some are low-grade and some advance into high-grade stages. Treatment differs according to which stage someone has. It is important to realize, however, that we currently have no medication to treat these dysplasias or the cervical cancers caused by HPV. All treatments involve some form of surgery.

Every year, 330,000 women develop a high-grade cervical dysplasia.[21] These women require more than simple Pap smears and gynecological exams. They need biopsies and surgeries. Another 1.4 million women acquire low-grade dysplasias, and they too need close monitoring, but not necessarily surgery.[22] Finally, about 4,000 women die from cervical cancer every year.

The causes of these dysplasias are various strains of HPV. We know that HPV types 16 and 18 cause 70% of all cervical cancers. These two also cause 50 to 60% of all high-grade dysplasias and about 25% of all low-grade dysplasias.

In addition to cervical cancer, HPV also causes genital warts. Strains 6 and 11 cause about 90% of all genital warts.

Physicians have witnessed the swell of HPV-associated pains over the past twenty years. Obstetrician-gynecologists have seen so much disease that many have become dulled to its presence, resigning themselves to the belief that there is little they can do to keep HPV under control. Sadly, many seasoned physicians have moved into a "damage control" mode, and simply tell young girls to try to make their boyfriends use condoms. The problem is, they know that this doesn't work. But is it the condoms? Don't kids listen? It is both. Condoms most certainly don't work well enough. And no, kids don't always listen, particularly when so few adults tell them the truth. Physicians feel outnumbered, outmaneuvered, and exhausted. Not infrequently, I have had young girls come to my office explaining that they were told that they had either an abnormal Pap smear test or early signs of cervical cancer, but had no idea how they contracted either. Their physicians see these problems so frequently that they simply forgot to tell them where the cancers came from.

While physicians buried themselves in work and teens watched television, listened to sex-infused song lyrics, and shopped for "sexy" clothes, those in medical research and development formulated a solid plan to combat cervical cancer and went to work. When Merck launched Gardasil, physicians and parents of fourth-grade girls were forced to confront the problem of young girls having sex. Many wondered if should they immunize their patients and daughters. Should they wait? Was this simply a money-making marketing maneuver?

Questions about the HPV vaccine opened furious debates among parents, doctors, educators, and even religious leaders. The problem really wasn't the vaccine. The problem was addressing sexual activity in young girls, coupled with the realization that the tried-and-true remedy (condoms) was no longer the panacea of old. Sex, cancer, and little girls. We had serious trouble on our hands.

The HPV vaccine covers only four strains of HPV: types 6, 11, 16, and 18. Remember, 16 and 18 cause 70% of all cervical cancers and, as best we know, the vaccine isn't 100% effective against those strains. So the vaccine certainly helps prevent cervical cancer, but it *only helps*. Like Dr. Gerberding said, the best way to prevent cervical cancer is to teach girls to wait as long as possible for their sexual debut, to reduce the number of sexual partners to as few as possible, and to avoid genital contact with another infected individual. (This last proposal is difficult, as 75% of the sexually active population has been exposed to HPV at one time or another.)

So in the mess of HPV infections, cervical cancers, cervical dysplasias, and genital warts, where are we left? My response is that we are left in a much more honest place. We know what we are dealing with and we know what to do. The problem, though, is this: are we willing to fight for what we know is right? We *can* slow the spread of HPV, and we *can* drive the numbers of cervical dysplasias and cancers down. The number of HPV-related problems wasn't always this high—and no, human feelings and desires weren't a whole lot different from what they are now. (Although one young fellow insisted after one of my lectures that we adults simply didn't understand their feelings. Middle-aged men, he continued, didn't experience sexual drives "back when they were teens" the way young men today do. Physiology, he insisted, had evolved.)

Teens have always wanted to have sex. The reason the STD epidemic exists *right now* is threefold.

First, kids are never told why and how to wait until they become sexually active. Parents, doctors, and teachers assume that kids will have sex early because they themselves did so as teens. These assumptions aren't prudent; they are cruel to kids. Second, our kids are trained to be sexually "on" at younger and younger ages. Third, an epidemic exists today that didn't exist 30 years ago. That's just the way it is, and we adults had better move out of the 1980s and into the twenty-first century.

Many parents wonder about the moral soundness of immunizing young girls against HPV. Again, this is more a medical issue than a moral one. Millions of men and women are infected with HPV, and if we can help young girls stave off cervical cancer, we must. Some argue that giving the vaccine sends the wrong message to girls. They believe that immunizing them gives them a green light for sexual activity.

This would certainly be a cruel message to give, particularly because Gardasil only helps reduce the risk of cervical cancer; it most definitely doesn't prevent it entirely. Also, HPV is only one of the many sexually transmitted infections girls risk contracting if they choose to be sexually active at an early age. The problems and pains associated with teens and sex reach far beyond HPV-associated problems.

I can't close the discussion about HPV without pointing out a schizophrenic irony. Here we are in the U.S. amid aggressive use of sex and sexual innuendo to advertise a multitude of goods to our young girls. We coerce our girls to act sexy, dress sexy, and engage in sexual activity. If we don't overtly encourage these personally, we watch as others do it to them. Then we take them to our pediatricians for annual physicals and have our daughters immunized against HPV and hepatitis B, both sexually transmitted. Can you imagine the outrage of conscientious, well-educated parents if we allowed aggressive marketing of cigarettes to our daughters and then took them to their doctors to be immunized against lung cancer? Clearly, no reasonable adult would stand for aggressive marketing of cigarettes to kids, knowing the harm smoking causes. Personally, I would rather my own kids smoke cigarettes during their teen years than have sex. If they smoke, they can quit and their lungs will heal. The long-term effects of smoking can be reversed if teens quit after three years. But if they were sexually active for the same three years, they could live with problems or infections that stay with them for life

Lydia's Story

Lydia became sexually active at 13. She was too scared to tell her mother or father and was even afraid to come in for her yearly physical. She was afraid that I would ask her if she was sexually active, and she didn't want to tell me. So, she just found excuses for not coming to the doctor. Finally, when she was 18, she had mononucleosis and had to come in. She was terribly sick with it. She had extreme throat pain, and her spleen and liver were affected. Because of her complications, I needed to follow her closely. As she recovered, we talked about her general health and she confided in me that she had been worried for the past five years that something was wrong with her. She had been having sex off and on over those years and had avoided pregnancy. But, she wondered, what else could she have? I told her that our conversations were confidential and that she needed a pelvic exam.

When she returned for one, I detected that indeed she had chlamydia, so I treated her with antibiotics and repeated her pelvic exam to be sure that it was gone. But I also found that she had an abnormal Pap smear. She had early cancerous changes in her cervix caused by HPV and she went right away to an obstetrician-gynecologist. There, she underwent a procedure called colposcopy. During the procedure, the doctor used a special magnifying instrument to look closely at her cervix. He took a biopsy of her cervical tissue to see how advanced the cancerous changes had become. Fortunately for Lydia, they weren't advanced, and she only needed close follow-up, which meant Pap smears every six months.

Having an abnormal Pap smear and being told that you have signs of cancer—no matter how early—is very hard for women. Many are scared, particularly young teens and those Lydia's age. And it's often embarrassing. Some doctors don't tell patients that cervical cancer is caused by an STD, simply because they don't want their patients to feel ashamed or embarrassed. Unfortunately, Lydia felt both ashamed and embarrassed. And worried.

There are different stages of cancerous changes, and the treatment chosen will vary depending upon the stage. A minimum of outpatient surgery is required to remove dangerous tissue. If cancer is advanced, a hysterectomy may be necessary. And of course, if the cancer has progressed beyond the cervix and uterus, chemotherapy and radiation therapy may be required. Remember, women *do* die of cervical cancer.

HERPES: THE RECURRING DREAD

Ever had a cold sore? Hurts, doesn't it? Imagine those cold sores on your genitals. Now you understand the devastation that the herpes virus wreaks. This virus is particularly nasty because it never disappears. It just goes "underground," hiding in certain nerve cells. It lies dormant there for months or even years until something—often stress—triggers an outbreak. Then the virus travels down the nerve out to the skin, causing ulcerated, painful lesions or blisters around your genitalia or your mouth. Obviously, you won't want to have sexual contact with anyone during an outbreak. But even when genital herpes lies dormant, you can still shed the virus, infecting sexual partners—or babies.

That's where its true danger lies. Babies infected by their mothers may become mentally retarded, suffer other brain damage, or become physically malformed. If a pregnant woman is infected, she may spontaneously abort or go into premature labor. The degree of risk to the baby is greatest if the mother experiences her primary herpes infection while pregnant. Delivering during such an outbreak means her baby has a 40 to 50% chance of becoming infected with neonatal herpes. And that means a 50% chance of death or permanent brain damage.[23] That's why obstetricians routinely perform cesarean sections in these cases. But like anyone else who carries the herpes virus, even when mothers don't have frank genital ulcers, they may still shed the virus and be contagious.

Erin's Story

"Dr. Warren, *please*, you've got to help us! It's Erin! She's turning blue! And her arms are flailing and shaking!" sobbed Angie into the phone. My partner, Dr. Warren, tried to calm the hysterical young mother, with little success. Finally, he convinced her to call 911 and tell the operator that her 3-day-old baby was having a seizure. He'd meet them at the emergency room.

When he arrived, he saw the tiny newborn lying still on the cold silver table. She was whitish gray, not pink, but at least she'd stopped seizing. As the emergency room doctor continued working with the baby, Dr. Warren turned to the parents. They could tell him nothing. Until the seizure, Erin had been a perfectly content baby. But a series of tests proved she was a very sick girl. Elevated white blood cell levels and abnormal glucose and protein levels indicated a viral infection. Twenty-four hours later Dr. Warren had a diagnosis: encephalitis—a potentially fatal brain infection resulting from the herpes type 2 virus circulating in Erin's spinal cord fluid, possibly in her brain tissue.

Erin's mother had told Dr. Warren that she never had any infections. "I don't have genital herpes," she insisted, when asked on several occasions during her pregnancy.

But her husband, Doug, *had* had a herpes infection as a teenager. Unfortunately, he had no idea the virus still lived in him, or that he'd passed it on to his wife, who, in turn, had passed it on to their new baby.

Erin was lucky. Unlike half of all babies born with herpes, she survived. But a brain scan taken when she was several weeks old showed damage to her brain tissue. Today, at age 3, she suffers from developmental delays. She walked late, talked late, and has a seizure disorder that requires daily medication. She'll be able to go to school, but we don't know how the disease affected her cognitive abilities, or what neurological problems await her in the future. We'll just have to see how she does over time.

What happened to Erin hit me hard. Teens have a choice about sex and STDs, babies don't. Erin paid a terrible price for what parts of our culture say is okay. Her father knows this, and lives every day confronted with the results of his carelessness.

It's no wonder physicians hate herpes. We hate how the virus attacks young children's bloodstreams and brains. We hate how difficult it is to treat. And we particularly hate its contagious nature.

Today, an estimated one in five Americans over the age of 12 is infected with herpes.[24]

Since researchers know that herpes is most frequently acquired during late adolescence and is rising fastest among our teens,[25] we must stop and ask ourselves how many millions of our kids are walking around with the virus who don't know they have it. Many people with the infection have mild symptoms or none at all.

When symptoms do appear, herpes behaves very differently from HPV in the body, causing a series of outbreaks. First comes the "primary" outbreak, usually resulting in a fever, generalized malaise, discomfort, and genital ulcers. This phase may last anywhere from 1 to 14 days. After the primary infection subsides, the herpes virus stays tucked inside nerve cells, waiting, until it erupts again. This subsequent eruption is called a "recurrent" or secondary outbreak. These are usually milder and less painful.

Although herpes often causes painful ulcers, many times patients have lesions without pain and don't recognize them as herpes. In fact, studies find that between 62 and 91% of those infected with the virus don't realize they have it.[26] They may miss a small sore that isn't painful, mistake symptoms of genital irritation or pain on urination for a bladder infection or allergic reaction, or suspect they're infected, but be too embarrassed to seek help.

That was the case with Anna. She got herpes when she was 15. At first, her mother thought she had a bladder infection and brought her in to see me. She had extreme pain when she urinated and a fever, and her whole body ached. She said she'd never felt such biting pain. The description of such intense pain led me to think that something more than a urinary tract infection was going on. As I examined her, I saw an ulcer on her labia. I asked how long she had had it. She said that she didn't know it was there. (She was typical of other teens who don't look at their genitalia.) I started her on acyclovir, a drug that causes the herpes virus to retreat from the skin or bloodstream into the central nervous system, where it lies dormant until the next eruption.

Together, Anna and I told her mother that she was sexually active and would live with herpes for the rest of her life. I reassured them that I would help Anna minimize outbreaks in the future, but even with drugs the painful lesions could recur.

Easy to Share

Herpes is considered more infectious than many other viruses. For example, it's much more communicable than HIV because less of it is needed to infect another person. While HIV is primarily transferred via body fluids, like semen and blood, herpes lives on the skin, as well as in body fluids such as vaginal secretions and saliva, all of which can transmit the virus.

We used to believe that the virus shed for only a few days after an infection or an outbreak, but studies show that herpes may shed *off and on for 8 to 10 years.* This means that a person with herpes can infect his or her sexual partner for a very long time. What complicates herpes infections is that while a person is shedding, he or she probably won't know it. In fact, 85% of all people who test positive for herpes shed the virus despite having no signs of clinical infection.[27] From a practical standpoint, this means that teens with the virus may infect future partners at any time because they (and their physicians) can't determine exactly when they're shedding.

Remember, this shedding occurs off and on, but the actual herpes infection stays in a person's body for life. Whether the person sheds the virus (i.e., is contagious) or not, he or she will continue to have genital outbreaks for the rest of his or her life. Shedding is different from the actual outbreaks themselves.

Sadly, the rising popularity of oral sex is an enormous contributing factor to the spread of herpes. Herpes can be as easily transmitted through oral sex as it can through vaginal sex. Signs of oral herpes include fever, pain on swallowing or eating, and ulcers in the mouth.

When herpes erupts on the skin or the lining of the mouth, it first appears as a small bump. Then it turns into a craterlike sore, or ulcer. The skin sends white blood cells to the area to fight the virus, and a yellowish crust forms. While the sore is still open, however, the virus is present. Whenever another person touches the sore, the virus spreads to the other person. Saliva quickly grabs the virus during oral sex and moves the particles around the mouth, resulting in oral herpes ulcers.

An Illness of Body and Mind

Because herpes is a lifelong disease, many people initially go through a grieving process when they're first diagnosed, moving through the stages of denial, anger, and grief, and finally into acceptance. Some become depressed, or so angry that they intentionally infect others in a misguided attempt to seek revenge. Victims report feeling like "lepers," outcast from their social groups. Others describe never feeling clean enough, or that they're "damaged goods." [28] Those with herpes also report plummeting self-esteem and a profound sense of loss. And studies find that about half of those with the disease suffer depression and rejection from their partners. About three-fourths say their enjoyment of sex drops; half say the spontaneity of sex disappears. [29]

Herpes is difficult enough for adults; it can be absolutely devastating for teens. Often, the teens I talk with say they'd give anything to be able to turn back the clock and begin again. At a time when teens feel too fat, stupid, short, tall, or awkward just being in the school cafeteria, dealing with herpes piles inordinate shame on top of already sagging self-esteem. Too often, these teens fall into deep depressions, which can be fatal if left untreated. You'll read more about this in Chapter 5.

HIV AND AIDS

I'll never forget the face of the beautiful 31-year-old woman who approached me after my lecture. Her eyes were avocado green and anxious. "Dr. Meeker," she began as she thrust her right hand forward into mine. "Thank you for telling these kids that sex is not a game. I began having sex as a teen, and in my early twenties I got HIV from a boyfriend. Now I have AIDS. Thank you, they need to know what sex can lead to down the road."

Of all the sexually transmitted diseases reported, it is fair to say that no disease is as frightening as AIDS. Although the disease is actually one of the least common sexually transmitted diseases in this country (an estimated 45,000 cases a year), [30] it is by far the deadliest. For African-American males between the ages of 15 and 44, AIDS is the leading cause of death. [31] That statistic points to the many changes in what was once thought of as a gay man's disease. It's now becoming a scourge among women as well. Between 1991 and 1995, the number of women diagnosed with AIDS increased by 63%, more than any other demographic group. And today, of the 900,000

people living with HIV in this country, 20% are women. Eighty percent of all transmission occurs sexually, not through injected drug
use or contaminated blood.[32]

As Harvey Elder, M.D., professor of medicine at Loma Linda
University School of Medicine in California, says: "We live in a toxic
and incestuous society—one that offers sex as the first choice remedy for all problems. When we fail to protect our youth from this
toxicity, we perpetuate HIV."

It's important to understand that while HIV can live in a variety
of body fluids, you can only become infected with HIV if you come
in contact with it in blood, semen, vaginal secretions, or breast milk.
The virus enters through the genital openings (anus and vagina),
through the mouth, through a break in the skin, or from mother to
infant through breast milk, or during pregnancy or delivery.

Dr. Elder teaches young doctors about HIV/AIDS, driving home
the message that the risk of HIV sexual transmission is directly
related to the number of sexual partners one has, as well as the
amount and type of sex one engages in.

Thus, he tells his students, if sexually active people limited new
partners to one every six months, HIV transmission would fall to
almost nothing. This is his own opinion, based on his own medical
practice, in which he treats dozens of HIV/AIDS patients a day, not
on any objective research. Perhaps it is a bit overstated, perhaps
not.

One problem with HIV is that you could have the virus and still
have a negative blood test. So many teenagers I care for may be
infected, but their symptoms won't show up until their 20s. *But it's
during the first several months after exposure that levels of the virus are
highest in blood, semen, and vaginal fluids, and thus most likely to be
spread.* That teens can spread the virus without realizing it scares me
to no end.

Treatment for teenagers is similar to treatment for adults. Treatment focuses on subduing the infection, vaccinating against other

infections, such as hepatitis A and B and pneumococcus (a bacterial infection), and watching closely for tuberculosis and other illnesses.

Unfortunately, the new medications used to treat AIDS have made us too relaxed about the seriousness of the disease, lulling many teenagers into complacency. When teenagers see basketball star Magic Johnson active and healthy, they come to feel that HIV is "no big deal." At times, I can't seem to get it into a teenager's stubborn head that HIV is not just an infection of homosexual men, but a disease that can ultimately kill them.

I wish they could see the mothers with AIDS whom I care for. See their anguish as they begin raising their young babies. These young women worry about *when*, not *if*, their disease will break out like a wildfire, killing them and orphaning their children. They can't breast-feed because their milk contains the deadly virus. They anxiously watch their baby's mouth for fungal infections. And every time their baby breathes too fast, mothers dread pneumonia—the result of a missed diagnosis. And they wait for their own breathing to go awry, signaling the same deadly sign. Their mental and emotional anguish is palpable. I've seen it. And that which causes their hearts to freeze with fear is entirely preventable. That's why I do my utmost to prevent this infection in *any* of my teen patients.

HEPATITIS B

Hepatitis B virus is a serious virus that can cause chronic infection, liver scarring, liver cancer, liver failure, and death. An estimated 4,000 to 5,000 people die each year in the United States due to the complications of cirrhosis and liver cancer as a result of hepatitis B. And an estimated 200,000 new hepatitis B infections occur each year.[33]

Besides the liver, the virus may damage the kidneys, blood vessels, skin, and joints. What many fail to realize is that hepatitis B is a sexually transmitted virus, present in blood, semen, saliva, and vaginal secretions. While infants and young children began receiving vaccinations against the virus in 1991, most of today's teenagers remain unimmunized. (In 1995, the National Advisory Committee on Immunization Practices recommended that immunization be extended to adolescents.)

Hepatitis B commonly occurs in adolescents and young adults. It can appear as an acute episode, in which the infection comes on quickly, causes serious illness, and then goes away. Or it can become a chronic illness, its victims living for many years with the residual effects of the disease, primarily liver damage.

The younger you are when the infection starts, the greater the likelihood that the infection will become chronic. Ninety percent of infants with hepatitis B develop the chronic disease, 60% of children under 5 develop it, and just 2 to 6% of adults with the acute infection will get chronic hepatitis B.[34]

Teens are considered a high-risk group for hepatitis B because 50 to 60% of transmission occurs through sexual activity. Gay teenage boys are at the greatest risk, as evidence suggests that one in five gay men are infected with hepatitis B.[35]

That's why it's highly recommended that sexually active teenagers (and homosexual men) receive the hepatitis vaccine. This is a series of three immunizations, shown to significantly reduce the likelihood of contracting the virus.

In fact, one reason we started immunizing infants was to ensure that, by the time they reached their teen years, they were protected. It's pretty difficult, as I've noted earlier, to get teenagers in to see doctors, let alone get them in for a shot. Infants are in the pediatrician's office several times a year.

Initially, hepatitis B symptoms include generalized malaise, nausea, diarrhea, abdominal discomfort, and perhaps a low-grade fever. But while hepatitis B may resemble the flu, it often doesn't go away like the flu does. We confirm the virus's presence with blood tests. Because we don't have any specific medications to kill the virus, treatment focuses on preventing and treating the complications and symptoms. For instance, intravenous fluids will treat the dehydration, while antinausea medicines will help with vomiting and nausea.

Many times the disease will go away on its own, but it may also go on to become chronic hepatitis. These patients will be chronic carriers of the disease. If a person has chronic hepatitis, he may suffer from mild or even severe liver problems. He may have pain that comes and goes, and his liver blood tests will be abnormal. But many others will simply be chronic carriers of hepatitis, without developing liver problems.

Hepatitis B is the most common sexually transmitted hepatitis, but it is not the only one. There is hepatitis A, which is transmitted through fecal matter and is more common among those who engage in anal intercourse. But there are also hepatitis C, hepatitis D, and hepatitis E. Although these are less common than A or B, they can be just as serious. Any infection that harms the liver is potentially life-threatening because the liver acts as a filter for the entire body. It both makes and breaks down different compounds in the body.

MORE STROKES

These are the broad, sweeping strokes of viral STDs. The nasty bugs may stay with us a lifetime. The ones I treat daily, the ones that come in dozens of forms, and the ones that our kids have to fight to prevent. This, however, is not the entire story. There's still another class of STDs that are new yet familiar at the same time, and that are presenting new problems that can't be overlooked.

FOUR

■ Nationwide, gonorrhea rates are highest among young women between the ages of 15 and 19.

Curable but Dangerous

BACTERIAL STDs. THEY HAVEN'T gone away. Their numbers are growing—especially among teens—and they're as dangerous, painful, and even as deadly as ever.

Bacteria and viruses are very different organisms. The most important difference is that you can stop bacterial STDs with antibiotics; this is not so with viruses. But bacteria are smart little germs, and when they're repeatedly exposed to many antibiotics, they mutate, "outsmarting" the antibiotic, becoming resistant to it. This has become a serious problem with the bacteria that causes gonorrhea, for instance.

Let's take a look at the most common bacterial STDs, and learn why they pose such a grave danger to our kids.

CHLAMYDIA

Chlamydia is the most commonly reported sexually transmitted disease in the United States. Thirty to 40%—nearly half—of the

3 million new cases each year occur in teens between the ages of 15 and 19.[1]

While health officials think its prevalence is declining in the general population, it continues to wreak havoc among teens. Teenage girls are most affected; about one in ten has the disease, compared with boys, in whom the numbers are closer to one in 20.[2] Just picture your daughter's soccer team. If all those girls are sexually active, at least one girl on that team is likely to have chlamydia. There are two primary reasons for the high numbers of chlamydia in teenage girls. First, about 85% of women and half of all men with the disease have no symptoms.[3] Because teens rarely see a doctor unless they're sick, it's hard to know if they're infected. And, of course, if they don't know they're sick, they can't be treated, and so they keep spreading the disease through sexual activity.

Second, chlamydia is hard to culture. When I perform a pelvic exam on a teenage girl, I take samples of cells from her cervix and vagina. I would pick up chlamydia only if the bacteria stayed in those areas. But sometimes, as the germ travels upward through the fallopian tubes and into organs beyond the uterus, it leaves the cervix. Thus, my cultures turn up negative for chlamydia, even though the girl is infected.

The only way to culture an infection in the uterus, fallopian tube, or any structure outside the uterus is through a surgical procedure called a laparoscopy, in which a gynecologist inserts a special instrument through an incision in the abdomen to examine the pelvic organs and take a tissue sample. This is a serious, invasive procedure, which we do not undertake lightly.

At first, the bacteria enters a girl's vagina and climbs toward the uterus, fallopian tubes, and ovaries. The primary symptoms are tenderness and a slight vaginal discharge. I always hope a girl has these symptoms, because then I might get to treat her early. But it's just as likely she won't know anything is wrong.

If chlamydia stays in a girl's cervix and doesn't spread, the disease lasts about 15 months and may clear up on its own. Other times, however, chlamydia spreads. Left untreated, chlamydia will cause PID in 20 to 40% of cases.[4] This results in severe abdominal pain, tenderness, and fever. If the chlamydia infection moves beyond a woman's reproductive organs into her abdominal cavity, it can cause scarring around her liver and diaphragm in a condition called the Fitz-Hugh and Curtis syndrome. It occurs in about 20% of young women with PID.[5] We can use antibiotics to heal the bacterial infection, but nothing can remove the scarring, which may result in chronic pain.

Once chlamydial infection develops into PID, infertility becomes a real threat. A startling one in four women with PID experiences problems such as ectopic pregnancy (pregnancy outside the uterus) or infertility.[6]

Infertility occurs in a variety of ways. The infection may scar a fallopian tube, and the scar tissue may block the tube. Since the fertilized egg travels along the fallopian tube to the uterus before implanting into the uterine wall to begin growing, this blockage would, effectively, stop any pregnancies. But in some instances, the fertilized egg can implant in the fallopian tube itself, causing an extremely dangerous condition called ectopic pregnancy. As the embryo grows, the tube eventually bursts and the young woman may die. Even if an infected woman is lucky enough to get pregnant, her baby is at risk of being born with eye infections and pneumonia.

Infertility is one of the most emotionally heartbreaking problems women can experience. And PID is one of the top reasons so many women experience infertility. Sadly, much of PID results from STDs acquired during the teen years.

Sandy's Story

I watched Sandy struggle with PID as a 17-year-old. She came to my office because she was having fits of abdominal pain that just wouldn't go away. She went to an urgent care center and the doctor told her she was experiencing severe constipation. He told her to go home and try some laxatives. She did. She came into my office three days later doubled over. When I examined her abdomen, she was in so much pain that she didn't even want me to touch her anywhere. When I told her that I needed to do a pelvic exam, I really believe she was so angry at me that she would have run out of the room if she could have.

When I performed the pelvic exam, she nearly jumped off the table when I moved her cervix. Her entire uterus was tender and inflamed, and I could tell just from examining her that the infection had moved into her fallopian tubes and was beyond her uterus. I took some cultures, which confirmed my suspicion of chlamydia, and admitted Sandy to the hospital so we could give her intravenous antibiotics. She responded well to the antibiotics and she behaved six months later as though she'd forgotten all about her experience. Sure enough, eventually she came back into my office with the same diagnosis and needed the same antibiotics. Repeat chlamydial infections are all too common in teens.

I was lucky enough to attend Sandy's wedding a couple of years later. She looked beautiful and excited, and married a terrific guy. As I watched her walk down the aisle, I felt a deep sadness. I knew what probably no one else at the wedding except Sandy knew. She was gorgeous and young and had so many years to look forward to. Would children be in her future? They could be, but the sad truth is, she markedly decreased her chances of having children because she had sex when she was too young. Chlamydia and PID change futures for way too many young women *and men*.

You see, chlamydia is gender-neutral, infecting men with nearly as much vigor. Although chlamydia does cause more damage in women, it harms boys as well, and 40% of males who are infected have no symptoms.[7] In males, the bacteria can result in infections of the internal genital organs, the epididymis, prostate, and urethra, making urination difficult. Fortunately, the disease doesn't cause infertility in men, and a course of antibiotics can wipe out the infection with no lasting effects. But an untreated infection may cause narrowing of the urethra or Reiter's syndrome, which causes conjunctivitis (an eye infection), infection of the urethra, arthritis, and unusual sores in the mouth. Chlamydia can also cause blood infections and arthritis in both men and women.

Frequently, I treat a patient for chlamydia only to see her return nine months later with another chlamydial infection. Why? Because often teens fail to change their sexual patterns even after they've had a wake-up call like an STD. This is a particular problem with an easily cured STD like chlamydia. Since a dose of antibiotics often clears up the infection, many young teens think it's no big deal and go right back to their risky sexual patterns.

GONORRHEA: BACK WITH A VENGEANCE

Gonorrhea used to be the good-news story on the STD front. While new diseases, including HIV, reared up in the 1980s and 1990s, rates of gonorrhea plummeted, thanks to intense public education, detection, and treatment campaigns on the part of public health officials. In the late 1990s, however, the disease bounced back. Now an estimated 650,000 cases are reported each year, and the actual number of gonorrhea infections is believed to be nearly twice that.[8]

But the statistic that most concerns me is this one: *Gonorrhea rates are highest among young women between the ages of 15 and 19.*[9]

One reason for the rising rates in adolescents may be the rising incidence of risky sexual behavior among teenagers. The more partners they have, the higher the risk of gonorrhea. And the wilder the sex (group sex, multiple partners in one night), the higher the rate of STDs. I'll discuss this in more detail in Chapter 9.

Gonorrhea is also a major cause of PID, infertility, ectopic pregnancy, and chronic pelvic pain in women. In women and men, gonorrhea can get into the bloodstream and cause septicemia and joint problems. Can you imagine a college senior with severe osteoarthritis? My colleague recently treated one.

Although patients are rarely hospitalized for arthritis, this young man was. Chip was 20 and had been sexually active since he was 15. He had tried heterosexual sex, then tried sex with men and liked it better. So he found one partner, then another, then more. Sometimes he used condoms, he said, sometimes he didn't. He had been treated for gonorrhea once, but it returned after he had sex with an infected man. He admitted that he didn't consider his first bout of gonorrhea "a big deal," since it was easily cured with antibiotics. But then he began having knee pain and fevers that came and went. When his knee became so swollen and painful he couldn't walk, he sought medical help. He didn't recall ever hurting his knee.

He was fortunate enough to see an astute physician who thought to take a sexual history. When the young man revealed his homosexuality, the doctor did a blood test and diagnosed the cause of his arthritis—the gonorrhea circulating throughout his blood. If he'd missed the infection and the disease remained untreated, at a minimum the bacteria would have continued to eat away at his knee joint, causing permanent damage. Or, the bacteria could have multiplied in his bloodstream, causing serious heart infection and perhaps death. In fact, in the era before antibiotics, gonorrhea caused 10% of all cases of endocarditis, an infection in the lining of the heart.

The young man was lucky. The intravenous antibiotics quelled the infection. Next time, however, he might not be so fortunate.

In the past few years, health officials have identified an alarming trend: increasing numbers of gonorrhea infections that are resistant to fluoroquinolones, the class of antibiotics typically used to treat them. Gonorrhea had become resistant to simple penicillin years ago. When bacteria like gonorrhea learn to outsmart antibiotics, there is only one thing to do: use stronger antibiotics. But it's only a matter of time before the bacteria outsmart *those* drugs.

So far, we've continued to win the race against antibiotic-resistant bacteria by coming up with more and more powerful medicines. But tucked in the recesses of many physicians' minds is the fear that there will come a time when medications can no longer stay one step ahead of the bacteria. Our medical armamentarium will be empty. The bacteria will win.

SYPHILIS INCOGNITO

The famous physician William Osler, M.D., once said, "He who knows syphilis, knows medicine." Syphilis is called "the great mimicker" because it can mimic the symptoms of virtually any disease, making it very difficult to diagnose. It is one of the oldest known STDs—its victims included Pope Alexander VI, Ivan the Terrible, and King Henry VIII. Unfortunately, these days its victims could include your niece or nephew.

Syphilis causes problems in men *and* women beyond the reproductive system. Left untreated, it advances through three stages. The first is called primary syphilis, in which a sore, or "chancre," appears on the genitalia. These ulcers are often hidden deep within the reproductive tract in women, who are usually unaware of them. The sore is not painful (like herpes sores can be) and usually clears up on its own even if not treated. But they increase the likelihood of sexual transmission of the HIV virus two- to fivefold.

If the patient doesn't recognize the sore and fails to get treatment, syphilis progresses to the secondary stage. The victim develops a rash of reddish-brown spots on the palms of his hands and the soles of his feet. The rash can also occur on other parts of the body. But it's identical to many other rashes, and so is often misdiagnosed. Again, even without treatment, the rash goes away on its own, but the syphilis bacteria remains in the body.

At the onset of the third stage, the bacteria attacks the heart, the nervous system, eyes, blood vessels, liver, bones, and joints. A person

with this late stage of syphilis experiences paralysis, numbness, difficulty coordinating his muscles, gradual blindness, and dementia.
Death is a very real possibility.

That's why it's so important that physicians diagnose syphilis as
early as possible in the course of the disease. With antibiotic treatment, syphilis can be stopped at either of the first two stages, thus preventing the final destruction of tissues and organs in the third stage.

Infected mothers can also pass the disease onto their babies.
Infants born with syphilis commonly have multiple, severe problems
of the brain and nervous system. They may have developmental
delays, seizures, and brain damage, and they often die. Nearly 25%
of pregnant women infected with the disease will miscarry.[10]

Years ago, as a pediatric resident working in a large inner-city hospital, I took care of a premature baby who began having seizures
shortly after birth. She was a big baby for 35 weeks—about 6
pounds. And she was beautiful, with clear, caramel-colored skin. We
successfully treated her seizures with an anticonvulsant. Although
her mother denied having any STDs, we knew better than to trust
her memory, so we tested the baby for syphilis. Her test came back
positive.

I felt sick. I knew when I saw the result that we were in for a hard
row. Sure enough, her seizures returned and got worse. We gave her
more and more medication and finally she developed intractable
seizures that medication couldn't affect. As the baby seized and
writhed I felt horribly helpless. We'd killed the bacteria in her blood,
but its effects on her brain were overwhelming. As her heart rate
slowed and we knew she was dying, we took her off life support and
I held her in my arms as the life in her flickered out. I wanted to take
her to her mother, but the woman said she couldn't hold the baby—
she was too distraught herself.

Syphilis had changed this family forever.

It is a horrible disease, but there is some good news on the syphilis
front. Rates of syphilis in this country are at their lowest levels ever,

and federal health officials have launched a plan to eradicate the disease entirely in the coming years. This disease is also less prevalent among teenagers; the highest rates are among women ages 20 to 29 and men ages 35 to 39.[11] That doesn't mean that sexually active teens never get this infection. They do, and it remains a serious danger. Gonorrhea rates had fallen a few years ago. Now they're back, stronger than ever. Syphilis may easily do the same.

TRICHOMONIASIS: HIV'S LITTLE HELPER

Trichomoniasis, a common STD in men and women, is caused by a parasite. It is not a bacterium, but we clump it with bacterial STDs because it responds to antibiotic treatment.

An estimated 5 million new infections occur each year, about one-fourth in teens (a very conservative estimate).[12] The organism that causes trichomoniasis has three tails and swims in the vagina, very much like sperm. Men usually have no symptoms, but some have burning with urination and ejaculation and a mild penile discharge. Some young women experience vaginal burning and itching and have a yellow-green frothy discharge, but 20 to 50% of women have no symptoms.[13] This makes the actual prevalence of trichomoniasis infection hard to establish. Additionally, even those women who *do* have symptoms often don't seek medical attention; they think the discharge and itching are due to menstrual problems or a yeast infection.

Left untreated, however, girls with trichomoniasis continue to infect their sexual partners, and have a higher risk of premature rupture of membranes during pregnancy and preterm delivery. One of the most serious problems with trichomoniasis is that it may increase the risk of HIV infection.[14] We don't really know why, since it doesn't generate the open sores of syphilis or herpes. Perhaps an immune system already stressed from fighting off the trichomoniasis can't effectively resist HIV.

Physicians treat trichomoniasis with oral medications such as Flagyl. However, the parasite has become increasingly resistant to treatment, and repeat courses of medication or higher doses are needed—sometimes delivered intravenously. As with any antibiotic-resistant bacteria, physicians fear that the trichomoniasis parasite may ultimately outsmart all our antibiotics.

BACTERIAL VAGINOSIS

Bacterial vaginosis is a very common infection in teen girls and women, often existing alongside sexually transmitted diseases. While it's not officially a sexually transmitted disease, it is, indirectly, caused by sexual activity. That's because sexual activity alters the balance of certain bacteria in the vagina, tipping the balance of good bacteria versus bad bacteria that normally reside there. This imbalance lets a harmful bacteria, called *Gardnerella vaginalis*, take over. The infection causes a grayish vaginal discharge with a fishy odor, and may occur even if a teen hasn't been sexually active.

Like trichomoniasis, bacterial vaginosis leads to far greater problems, increasing the risk of PID and HIV infection. In pregnant women, the disease leads to premature births and low-birth-weight babies.

MY PATIENTS ARE YOUR CHILDREN

I remember a young teenager who died in the emergency room when I was a second-year pediatric resident. I'd failed to see that she was experiencing a fatal drug overdose, and thought she had an infection. She just didn't *look* like my perception of what a drug addict looked like. Another physician reprimanded me after she died. "Didn't you do a drug screen?" he asked in amazement.

"I just didn't think about it," I said.

"You can't afford *not* to think about it," he said. "These kids' lives depend on you."

I will never forget his words. Today they apply to this new epidemic, which we cannot ignore or refuse to think about. Failing to recognize this epidemic for what it is could kill our kids just as surely as that drug overdose took the life of that young woman.

Now that you've met some of my patients and seen a slice of the world I see every day, look around. My patients are just like your kids, your nieces and nephews, the teens at church with you on Sunday morning, at football practice, and at piano recitals. They are the potential victims of this epidemic.

In the following pages, you'll learn about another epidemic—one that is gaining momentum and that proves to be as dangerous and perhaps even more painful than viruses and bacteria.

FIVE

■ Suicide is the third leading cause of death among young people ages 15 to 24.

The Emotional STD

AS A DOCTOR, I CAN PROBE, CULTURE, prescribe antibiotics, and aggressively treat and track contagious STDs. But depression is different. It's more elusive, yet equally, if not more, dangerous. It can come and go, or it can settle in, making itself so comfortable in an adolescent's psyche that it's nearly impossible to extricate. There, just as many STDs do, depression causes permanent damage that may not become apparent for years. To many teenagers, depression can make them feel as though another entity has moved into their body, taking over everything they think, feel, and do.

For the thousands of teens I've treated and counseled, one of the major causes of depression is sex. I consider it an STD with effects as devastating as—if not more—HPV, chlymadia or any other.

Just ask any doctor, therapist, or teacher who works closely with teenagers and they'll tell you: Teenage sexual activity routinely leads to emotional turmoil and psychological distress. Beginning in the 1970s, when the sexual revolution unleashed previously unheard-of sexual freedoms on college campuses across the country, physicians began seeing the results of this "freedom." This new permissiveness, they said, often led to empty relationships, to feelings of self-contempt and worthlessness. All, of course, precursors to depression.

Teens are particularly vulnerable to the negative effects of early sexual experience because of the intense and confusing array of emotions they're already experiencing. Adding sex to the picture only makes those feelings more intense and more confusing.

Like most STDs, depression remains hidden and underdiagnosed, even though its prevalence among our teenagers has skyrocketed in the past 25 years, paralleling the rise in STDs. We don't know exact numbers because so many of its victims can't put a name to their feelings, while too many adults pass off depressed behavior in teenagers as part of "normal adolescence." Other teenagers are so depressed they lack the energy or desire to seek help. For while physical pain drives patients to physicians, emotional pain keeps them away.

SKYROCKETING RATES

Still, the numbers we do have on depression in teens are terrifying. According to Dr. John Graydon, professor of Psychiatry and Neurosciences at the University of Michigan, one in eight teenagers is clinically depressed and most teens' depression goes undetected.[1] Because the rates of completed suicides among adolescents have skyrocketed 200% in the past decade,[2] suicide now ranks as the third leading cause of death in teenagers, behind accidents and homicides[3] (both of which may involve depressed adolescents, who often drink and engage in violent behavior to anesthetize their depressed feelings).

Also frightening is the fact that teens today are more likely to succeed in killing themselves when they try. One study found that completed suicides among 10- to 14-year-olds increased 80% from 1976 to 1980 and 100% for 15- to 19-year-olds.[4] From 1980 to 1997, the rate of suicide increased 11% in all 15- to 19-year-olds, 105% in African-American teen boys, and a startling 109% in 10- to 14-year-old children.[5] Even more sobering is the fact that for every adolescent who succeeds in committing suicide, 50 to 100 attempt it.[6] In fact, a 1995 study found that a staggering 33 out of every 100 high school and middle school students said they'd thought of killing themselves.[7]

One-third of our adolescent population has thought of killing themselves!

This statistic terrifies me, as it does countless parents, teachers, and grandparents in the country. Indeed, many experts on adolescent suicide and psychiatric illness refer to this dramatic increase as "a national tragedy."[8] And I strongly believe, as do many of my colleagues, that the situation is much worse, that depression is highly underdiagnosed in teens. The bottom line is that depression has invaded millions of our teens. And that's just what we see on the surface.

I believe even more strongly that there is a correlation between the explosion in sexual activity and the epidemics of STDs and depression in our teenagers. I know this because of what I've heard from the thousands of teens I've counseled over the past 20 years, and from my own experiences raising four children. What I hear and see is that sexual freedom causes most of them tremendous pain. Now, research is just beginning to show a correlation between teen sex and STDs. One study shows such a strong link between STDs and depression that the authors advised all physicians to screen every teen with an STD for depression.[9] I go one step further—I screen all sexually active teens for depression, STD or not.

We already know that adults with STDs struggle with depression, guilt, and feelings of isolation and shame. And we know from several significant research studies that the breakup of teenage romantic relationships often leads to depression and alcohol abuse. One study of 8200 adolescents, ages 12 to 17, found that those involved in romantic relationships had significantly higher levels of depression than those not involved in romantic relationships.[10] "Something about dating and dating relationships can be toxic to girls' health," says Susan Nolen-Hoeksema, Ph.D., a psychology professor at the University of Michigan in Ann Arbor, and an expert in adolescent depression.[11]

Darlene's Story

Consider Darlene, a 17-year-old patient of mine who sank into a deep depression after her first sexual encounter with her ex-boyfriend. I first met Darlene when her parents brought her in because they were concerned about her behavior. She came at their prompting, but also because she, too, felt she needed help. This is unusual. Most teens (even depressed ones) are dragged in by their parents; few come of their own accord.

During that first visit, I spoke with her and her parents together. Darlene said she preferred that her parents stay in the room at the beginning of our discussion. I was pleased about this, because that showed she had a healthy, open relationship with both of them.

I learned during that first appointment that Darlene had broken up with her boyfriend of two years because she felt, as she said, that she'd "outgrown the relationship." After a one-month hiatus, she visited him on an impulse. They began talking and, ". . . before I knew what was happening, we were having sex." Afterward, she said, she was furious with him, but even more angry at herself. I asked why she felt so angry at herself. She said she'd promised herself that she only wanted to have sex in a deeply felt, meaningful relationship, and that this encounter had happened without much thought or feeling, with someone she had already broken up with. She felt she'd let herself down. "And I didn't even like him that much," she said, crying. I was touched to see her father reach out and hold her hand.

At the time, Darlene had told her mother what happened, and together they went to a local pregnancy counseling center where a blood test confirmed she wasn't pregnant. A few days later, she told her father what had happened and he, too, responded with great sensitivity and compassion. "My mom and dad have been incredible," said Darlene. "I just don't get why I'm so upset. They didn't yell at me or anything. They've just been loving me. I can't believe I was so stupid."

But in the weeks after the incident, Darlene began withdrawing from both her parents and her friends. She became angry easily. She slept during the day and stayed up late at night—all unusual patterns of behavior for her. She even wanted to drop out of the basketball team, her favorite sport. When her parents saw Darlene's behavior worsen rather than improve, they brought her in to see me.

During that first visit, I confirmed their suspicion that Darlene was seriously depressed. I hooked her up with a good counselor, but still saw her weekly for the next few months to make sure her depression was lifting. During these months, I realized that Darlene's depression resulted from unresolved grief related to a deep sense of loss. Loss of her virginity, her self-respect, her parents' respect, her sense of control over her behavior, and her commitment to herself. She felt so overwhelmed by these losses she didn't know how to process them and bring them to resolution.

Even though her parents said they forgave her, she didn't believe them. How could they forgive her when she couldn't forgive herself?

Many advocates of sexual freedom among teens would argue that she was overreacting. They would say that her real problem was that she valued her virginity and her commitment to it too much. They would say that her parents set her up for depression because they didn't teach her that sex is normal for kids her age. That if she would only accept this "reality," she wouldn't feel any real losses. Finally, they would insist she has nothing to forgive herself for, because she didn't do anything wrong. And that this is a lesson her parents should have taught her.

But there's no arguing with a person's feelings. I believe Darlene's feelings needed to be acknowledged by an adult whom she respected and to whom she listened. That's exactly what her counselor, parents, and I did over the next months. We helped her recognize her losses, validate them, and grieve them one at a time. Then we worked to help her to forgive herself. As she resolved each loss and forgave herself, her depression lifted and her "normal" life returned.

Darlene was lucky. She got help before her depression dragged her down so deep she drowned in it. Millions of kids never get that help.

Searching for Proof

Given stories like Darlene's, why doesn't research yet exist linking depression to teenage sexual activity? Three reasons.

First, these twin epidemics have come upon us so quickly there simply hasn't been time to conduct the studies. But I don't need to wait for formal studies to affirm what I already see—and my observations are not isolated ones. At pediatric conferences many of my colleagues report the same thing: increased post-traumatic stress disorder in sexually active teens.

I also make the link between sex and depression when I look at our world today from a bird's-eye view. Consider that life in the United States is relatively stable, with a historically high level of economic abundance. Why should our children be so depressed? And why should so many of them be thinking of killing themselves? Consider the words of Armand Nicholi, M.D., a professor of psychiatry at Harvard Medical School, and an expert on adolescent psychiatric problems: "When future historians study American culture, . . . they may find it perplexing and paradoxical that during an era of unprecedented leisure time and prosperity, millions of adolescents used psychoactive drugs to alter their feelings and to escape their environment. That each year, during an era of unprecedented openness and frank discussion of sexuality, hundreds of thousands of unmarried teenagers became pregnant and experienced an abortion; and that during an era of unprecedented scientific discovery and opportunity, thousand of adolescents both attempted suicide and succeeded in killing themselves." [12]

Second, in order to conduct studies on the link between teen sex and depression, we would have to start with the hypothesis that, perhaps, indeed there is a link—something that many funding institutions are not willing to do because it opposes more liberal views about teen sex. It's difficult, if not downright unpopular, today to take a stand that questions whether sexual freedom is good or bad for teenagers.

Third, there's a great deal of money at stake. If solid research finds that sexual activity in teens leads to depression, it would force many businesses to take a hard look at advertising and the media in general. Businesses would need to look at how sex is used to sell products to the teen demographic group, which today has perhaps the largest buying influence in the history of our economy. To put it simply, the business of selling to teens relies on sexual messages.

We have more experts, more research, and more sophisticated antibiotics, antivirals, and antidepressants than ever before in the history of our country. We understand psychological illness, adolescent behavior, and parenting strategies, yet we've never had as many depressed teens and adolescents as we do today. Why is depression so rampant? Why is teen suicide exploding to the point that it's called a national tragedy? Because our teenagers are hurting and are lonelier than ever before, and because so many stimuli encourage them to find solace for their loneliness and hurt through sex. This doesn't take their hurt away, it only makes it worse.

Tony's Story

Tony is a 14-year-old patient of mine who isn't sure if he's gay, straight, or bisexual. So he asked *me* what *I* thought he was. Interestingly, he asked me this without giving me any information about his sexual feelings. (Many kids believe that I have some magical insight into who they are, what they feel, how many sexual partners they've had, and what their sexual orientation is, even before they tell me anything.) I said I didn't know, and suggested he tell me his thoughts about sex.

Tony said he'd never really had sex. Well, I know that today's kids have different ideas about what constitutes sex, so I asked him about certain sexual behaviors—oral sex, mutual masturbation—and he shook his head at all of my queries. However, I did learn that he was involved with online chat rooms, in which the conversations were very sexual. They talked about sex and having sex with girls, guys, and those who claimed to be bisexual, using erotic, explicit language that stimulated Tony. But Tony was puzzled because he became just as sexually excited by exchanges with boys as with girls. He started downloading pornography online. Some were pictures of guys, some of girls. Some showed heterosexual sex, some homosexual sex.

Shortly after he started viewing this pornography, he began having sleep difficulties. He had dreams in which he had sex with girls, men, women, and boys, performing all sorts of acts. He became agitated around friends at school and, at soccer practice one day, had a panic attack "out of the blue." He didn't want to shower with his team after practice. He didn't want to go to sleep at night for fear of his dreams. He said he couldn't tell his parents because they would think he was a "freak." So he figured the best solution was to come to his doctor and find out what he "was." If he knew, his nightmares and panic attacks might go away, he reasoned.

Tony's problem clearly had nothing to do with his sexual orientation. He was struggling from a mild form of post-traumatic stress disorder precipitated by his exposure to cybersex and pornography. He experienced normal sexual arousal when he viewed pictures and sexual language. Because of his age and concrete-thinking style, he believed that because he was aroused by men and women he was either gay or bisexual. This caused him further confusion and trauma, not to mention anxiety. But what really caused this anxiety was not his sexual arousal, but his exposure to deeply disturbing adult material.

The association of healthy, normal arousal with traumatic pictures and language left him confused and anxious. We decided to deal with the real issue at hand, and worry about his sexual orientation later. Once we sorted out that the pornography and cybersex were the problem, not his sexual orientation, his anxiety and nightmares resolved. This brought him great relief.

SEX AND DEPRESSION

Sex and depression present a kind of chicken-and-egg conundrum. Studies find that kids who are depressed gravitate toward sex, since sex acts as a drug, numbing a hurt, filling a void, keeping their minds altered, if only for a moment. But sexual activity also leads to depression.

It's important here to understand the psychological roots of depression. In teens, depression is a prolonged state of grieving. Normally, one goes through a series of stages in resolving grief: denial, bitterness, anger, sadness, and acceptance. But if, for some reason, you experience hurt or loss and you *don't* go through this grieving process, depression can result.

For instance, a teenage boy may feel terrible sadness because he just broke up with his girlfriend, but he doesn't allow himself to exhibit that sadness for fear that someone (mom or dad perhaps) will notice and make fun of him. Or an adolescent girl who had sex and now feels guilty and confused may not allow herself to acknowledge these emotions, pushing them deep inside where they fester into depression.

This refusal to grieve takes the form of an unpeeled onion. The outer layer is denial that there is any problem, loss, or hurt. This is the most visible layer, and is obvious when teenagers insist I've got them figured all wrong, that they aren't depressed.

Beneath this layer of denial lies bitterness and anger. This anger stems from a sense of loss, and, as we'll see later, there are numerous losses associated with sex. For instance, there is the loss of self-respect.

Even if a teenager is mature enough to recognize this loss, if he doesn't move past the stage of anger to sadness, where he can grieve this loss, he may become "stuck" in anger at himself.

Or a teenage girl may experience loneliness and a feeling of betrayal after a sexual relationship. If she fails to grieve those feelings properly, she may turn her hurt and anger inward, becoming "stuck" in persistent, unresolved anger and exhibiting harmful behavior, lashing out, stealing, engaging in self-destructive behavior (sex, drugs, alcohol). It may look like rage, but it is also depression.

One classic example of how kids turn this rage inward is the preponderance of body piercing. Punching holes in intimate parts of their bodies, such as their lips, tongue, belly button, or even vagina, sends a message to the world: "I am hurting this intimate part of myself because I don't like who I am." When girls pierce the sexual parts of their bodies, their labia and nipples (some so severely they'll never be able to nurse a baby), they're saying: "I am cutting on my womanhood. This is anger turned upon the self."

Beneath this anger often lies sadness. It's much safer and easier to feel the anger, I tell teens, than it is to feel this sadness. Anger lets energy out, whereas sadness only consumes energy. When you're sad, you want to be comforted, and too many teens have no one to comfort them. So they keep their sadness to themselves. The hurt stays like a crusted-over abscess on their hearts. Then they become angry with themselves because they're sad (irrational, yes, but this is teenager thinking), and angry with their family and friends because no one will help them get rid of their sadness or their anger.

At the center of this onion of depression is a hole—the empty space left when that which was so precious and prized is taken away. And, as you'll see, much is lost when teenagers have sex before they're ready. These losses are substantial, and can be devastating to the teenage soul.

Loss of self-respect. While many teenage boys claim sex is fun, just as many admit (if given the opportunity) that they lose respect for themselves after a sexual encounter. Some may boast about their sexual exploits and appear on the outside to have gained self-confidence. But others admit to me in private that something changed inside them after they started having sex. They have less self-respect, having given up their sexual intimacy to someone they didn't care deeply about. Many also struggle with the feeling of loss of control during sex—control of their emotions and control of their bodies. Some teens become annoyed with their female partners for having so much influence over their emotions. Other boys don't like losing physical control of their bodies during orgasm. Experiencing an orgasm may be embarrassing, particularly if they don't know the girl well. She may make fun of his penis or ejaculate, or they're left open to criticism for premature ejaculation, which can be emotionally traumatic. With one disgusted look, a girl has the power to slice his manhood in two. This can have devastating effects on teenage boys, who need a healthy view of their masculinity.

Girls have the potential to feel an even greater loss of self-respect. Part of the problem is that American girls are at times poorly versed in setting physical boundaries. They've at times failed to learn to protect their bodies. They're encouraged to expose every inch of skin they can get away with (think Britney Spears). In doing so, girls are taught that their bodies are not worth protecting. Self-respect issues arise when a girl feels that she's surrendered control of her body to her sexual partner. If her partner fails to receive what she gives with the respect and awe it deserves, she feels hurt, disappointed, embarrassed, and cheated. When she turns these feelings inward upon herself, the end result is depression.

Loss of virginity. I believe that protecting one's virginity is hardwired into our psyches, much as self-preservation is. We don't train ourselves to respond this way, we are born with it; it's part of our "fight or flight" response. I believe that preserving our virginity is one part of what we are naturally conditioned to protect, because I have witnessed hundreds of teens grieve the loss of their virginity.

Intuitively they know that their virginity is something special. It is private and it is deep.

Proof of the unique and valuable nature of one's virginity can be seen in kids who are sexually abused. Every young child, adolescent, and teen I have cared for who has been sexually abused hates talking about it. Psychologists and psychiatrists universally accept the fact that most kids who have been sexually abused won't readily admit that sexual violation has occurred. Teens will admit when their feelings have been hurt or if they have been physically hit, but they don't want to admit to sexual violation. Why? Because their virginity and their sexuality are separate from their feelings or their bodies. Virginity is more special.

Think about this for a moment. If a girl didn't value her virginity highly or feel that it was unique, why wouldn't she openly discuss it? The very fact that something extremely precious has been taken away or violated is one of the reasons kids of all ages keep sexual abuse a deep, dark secret. And the fact that lifelong pain ensues when sexual boundaries are crossed, or when virginity is wrenched from a child in a manner that makes her feel helpless, gives testimony to the incredible value of virginity.

Some might argue that losing one's virginity voluntarily, as with teen sex, falls in a different category. Certainly it does. But the inherent value of virginity remains the same. If a teen surrenders it voluntarily, she knows that she has given a part of herself that occupies a place of extraordinary prominence in her being. So even when a teen surrenders virginity voluntarily, the loss is still great. And it is still deep.

Finally, many teens want to protect their sexual innocence. This desire stems from a natural one to keep oneself separate, to erect healthy boundaries around one's body. Teens want privacy—private conversations, private thoughts, private behaviors. This is natural and it is intuitive. So, too, is their sense of privacy surrounding their sexuality. And at the core of this sexuality is their virginity.

But in the midst of the flood of sexualized messages from media, this natural mechanism of privacy preservation is broken down. These media messages train teens to tear down healthy boundaries to their privacy, their sexuality, and their virginity. This can cause tremendous distress and even depression for teens.

Loss of trust. Unless teens have sexual encounters strictly as a form of "fun," it's quite possible they may lose trust in their partners. They may begin sex because it is fun, but realize afterward that it involves much more serious feelings than they anticipated. For whenever teenagers expose private parts of themselves (emotionally or physically) during sex, they are exhibiting great trust in their partner. If this results in a pleasant experience, their trust grows, but if it ends badly, their trust is destroyed.

For instance, during sex, a boy may tell a girl she's lousy, fat, or inexperienced. When this happens, her trust in him that he will make a very serious encounter "safe" is destroyed. Trust is also harmed when teenagers spontaneously end sexual relationships for seemingly no reason, or when they see their partners moving on to other sexual relationships. Or when they hear gossip in the halls about private moments they shared with another.

This loss of trust after the intimate experience of sex can be emotionally devastating. Think about it. Teenagers often seek out sex because they need another person to respond to them consistently, with positive feedback. Take the teenage boy, for instance, who is athletically clumsy, perhaps kind of nerdy. He hesitates to let even his parents see his real feelings because he fears they will ridicule him. He tries to protect himself (quite reasonably) by staying quiet. But he desperately wants and needs to know if he's got a normal masculinity.

The best way to find out, he reasons, is to have sex with a girl. So he tries it. When he does, he is, in essence, "showing" her his masculinity, strutting before her like a male robin preens and struts before his mate. When she fails to applaud him for his sexual prowess, the shape of his body, etc., then the trust he placed in her is lost. She blew it, just like all the rest, not giving him what he needed, letting him down. Since he's so egocentric, he reasons that the problem must be with him, not with her. Since she let him down, he really *is* a jerk and a nerd. He pushes those feelings deep inside him, where they fester, leading to depression.

Loss of expectations. As seasoned researcher and psychiatrist Helene Deutsch wrote in the 1960s, when the sexual revolution was just taking off, adolescents "suffer from emotional deprivation and a kind of deadening as a result of their so-called free and unlimited sexual excitement. . . the spasmodic search for methods by which to increase the pleasure of the sexual experience indicates unmistakably that the sexual freedom of our adolescents does not provide the ecstatic element that is inherent—or should be—in one of the most gratifying human experiences." [13] Once they find the sexual experience doesn't meet their expectations, she goes on to say, teens all too often turn to drugs and show an increasing interest "in sexual perversions," resulting in what she refers to as the rise of "psychological disaster" in teens.

I call it the result of smashed expectations. For quite often, teenagers build up the sexual experience in their minds, expecting it will fill their emptiness while meeting their needs for love and acceptance and belonging. For instance, teens often use sex as a way to fill the void of loneliness that results from a broken family. All too often, however, those expectations are never met, leaving teens with a grinding emptiness, resulting in frustration, agitation, and depression.

I saw this happen to Andrew when he was 16. He'd been my patient for several years. His mother brought him in because she suspected he was depressed. His grades had dropped and he didn't want to go to school. Andrew was a talented artist, and his mother noticed that the drawings scattered around his bedroom had dark and gruesome themes. As I began treating Andrew for his depression, he revealed that ever since his father left the family when he was 6, he worried about his mother. "She cries a lot," he said, and this upset him terribly.

His father was basically absent, and his refusal to send Andrew's mother money to help pay for his clothes, books, and expenses also upset the boy. Sometimes the father called, sometimes he didn't. Andrew never knew what to expect. "I just wish my dad would disappear for good," he said angrily, fighting back tears. The relationship, such that it was, just hurt too much.

When he was 11, Andrew said, an older boy had raped him. The experience left him confused, embarrassed, ashamed, and too afraid to tell anyone. After that, he said, he distanced himself from other boys, preferring the company of girls. At 14, he began having casual sex with girls. "I needed to figure myself out," he said. Was he gay or was he straight?

But I could see past that. I knew that by having sex with girls, Andrew was really trying to find acceptance of his masculinity, relief from his loneliness, and, quite simply, some love and affection. It was so obvious to me, because when he described what he wanted from sex, he suddenly jumped to talking and crying about his father. About how he was never around. About how disappointed his father must be in him, because otherwise his dad would come around more. Now he was sobbing about how desperately he wanted his dad. His body language regressed, he drew his knees to his chest and hugged them. Then he began asking me over and over why his father did that. "Did what?" I asked.

"Why did he hurt us so bad? What did I do wrong? Why did he leave us?" Suddenly I realized that Andrew was back in his house watching his father pack his things and leave. The tears and facial expressions made me understand that he was in excruciating pain. There it was. The center of the onion of depression, the layers peeled away. He wanted his dad back. He wanted his hugs, his voice, his affirmation that he, Andrew, was okay. Sex, in his mind, was a way to get those things he'd never received from his father.

But sex never delivered. It only made him crazy and eventually depressed. Why? Because Andrew lives in a culture that teaches him that sex is pleasurable, exciting, and full of promise. But the reality is vastly different. In my experience, it's far more disappointing and frustrating to teens than it is pleasurable. In fact, I've asked hundreds of teenage girls whether or not they like having sex, and I can count on one hand those who said they did. Once they confront their smashed expectations, many teenagers feel something is wrong—not with sex itself, but with themselves. So they try harder to make sex "work," to make sex provide those things they think it should: intimacy, love, trust, acceptance, appreciation of their masculinity or femininity, relief from their loneliness. When it doesn't work, millions of teenagers, like Andrew, assume something is wrong with *them*, and turn their anger and hurt inward, resulting in depression.

Andrew was able eventually to understand his feelings and his behavior better. The process took several months, but he learned that sex couldn't give him what he needed from his dad. To the contrary, it only crushed his sense of self-respect and self-worth. But he also learned he could work on developing good male friendships to alleviate his loneliness. When that happened, he found his sexual desire diminished. He still wanted it, he said, but he didn't "need" it. He was experiencing healthy sexual desire outside of emotional voids.

Freud called this cycle repetition/compulsion, in which we repeatedly return to certain behaviors such as sex, drugs, or drinking to get something that continually eludes us. When we feel empty, we return to a place in which we hope to find some relief or satiation of our desires or needs. Even when our behavior fails to satisfy those needs, we return again and again, trying harder to find what doesn't exist.

This is what teenagers often do, turn again and again to sex, hoping to find something that doesn't exist, sinking deeper and deeper into depression.

THE SPECIAL LOSS OF DIVORCE

One of the greatest losses our teenagers feel is the loss inherent in divorce. When parents divorce, children experience both the physical loss of a parent and the concurrent feelings of abandonment and lack of control. Some teens can handle the death of a parent better than they do a divorce. At least, they rationalize, there is no choice in death.

As I've seen in my practice time and time again, divorce loss often propels kids into early sex. Let me explain.

We've seen this situation feebly played out on television countless times: Teens feel a large, undue responsibility for the divorce of their parents. It matters not how many times their parents reassure the teen that he or she is not responsible for the divorce. It's part of how a teen's mind works. A teenager's own adolescent self-centeredness and sense of power will negate rational thought, leaving him with pure emotion. As these losses accumulate, some require serious grieving.

Teens who have a good support system and a strong sense of connection with their parents or other adults are able to grieve losses to resolution. They allow themselves to feel their sadness, anger, and hurt, and even talk about them to friends and adults if they believe that their feelings will be respected.

Healthy parents are crucial to this process. We are the ones who provide the safe environment in which teens can feel and resolve their emotions. We need to be on the lookout for losses that occur in our children's lives so we can help them work through loss and resolve their hurt feelings.

But too often, teens suppress their emotions because they are simply too afraid to let them show at home. As children in our society grow into adolescence, they experience the loss of a sense of being protected, loved, and cared for.

Let's face it, too many teens are ignored in our culture. Within their own community, it seems everyone is too busy for them. Sometimes their doctor barely has time to talk to them; often both parents work and are too tired to talk when they come home; teachers are stretched thin by overcrowded classes; and psychiatrists have three-month waiting lists. I believe this generation of teens is the loneliest generation in the history of our country. Some parents push them away with the excuse that their kids need to become independent and world-savvy, when, in fact, parents just want their own lives. Kids require energy and patience, which many parents are often too tired to provide.

Too often, kids have no one with whom to figure out life, no one with whom to communicate their anger, sadness, or even the emptiness that life can bring. For teens to acknowledge that they never felt genuinely loved, never experienced healthy intimacy with a parent, and that no one of significance in their life really values them, would cause their world to cave in. Thus, they stuff it. They get stuck in depression. The onion stays unpeeled, an abscess at the center of their soul, waiting quietly for someone to prick it open and drain it.

That's when teens turn to sex, an action that relieves the momentary isolation, but which often leads to more loss in an endless cycle of emotional angst.

THE TRIUMVIRATE OF DEPRESSION

When I counsel teens who are depressed, I try to help them view themselves as whole people who have three dimensions—physical, psychological, and spiritual. I often explain that depression may start in one dimension and then spread to another.

The physical roots of depression generally stem from low levels of various neurochemicals, such as dopamine, norepinephrine, and serotonin. These chemicals play critical roles in the areas of energy, emotions, sensations, and cognition. Nerve endings in the brain release these chemicals, also called neurotransmitters, and they circulate throughout brain tissue until other nerve endings take them back up, similar to the way you suck up soda through a straw. If they aren't released in sufficient amounts, or are taken up too quickly before the brain has a chance to use them, depression can result.

I try to explain to teens that these physiological changes are completely real and completely out of their control. Just as someone with diabetes suffers from low levels of insulin, those with depression have altered levels of neurochemicals. No one asks for diabetes, no one asks for depression. Sometimes it just happens.

Serious depression can be caused by these imbalances, and for these types of illnesses, drug therapy is often the answer. But for the majority of physically healthy teens, this is not the cause. And unless I see clear signs of acute, long-term depression, we don't go the drug route.

The second dimension I talk about is the psychological, which I described earlier as "peeling back the onion." It's the layers of our subconscious, and as they emerge, these layers define who we are. In the case of depression, our psychological well-being depends greatly on how we handle denial, bitterness, anger, and other emotions as we move toward acceptance of difficult losses. This, as you've likely noticed, is a big part of the counseling I do.

What I haven't talked about yet is the spiritual component. I believe that addressing spirituality for teens is good medicine. And I address it here because the depression that comes from the losses teens feel that are associated with sex are similar to those associated with spirituality. In other words, sex is a spiritual experience.

Spirituality and Depression

Teaching teens that there is a dimension of life that we cannot see is easy. Intuitively, they get it. They know that they are deeper than just flesh and bones, and they appreciate it when an adult affirms this. In fact, one of the most delightful aspects of talking with teens is hearing them develop deeper and more abstract thinking. They wonder out loud about the meaning of life and the existence of God. When I ask them about spiritual issues, most love talking about it. It makes them feel smart and adultlike. So I probe and ask questions and they open up.

Most teens admit they believe in a god, either because of upbringing at home or through their church. They have an involvement, a relationship with a "Father above." Teenagers like the idea of being able to trust in a higher being when they experience difficulty doing things on their own. God becomes their safety net, their power source, the one who takes over when they mess up. I've treated many really troubled teens who straightened out their lives and discovered and developed an abiding relationship with God, in whatever way each individual teen perceives this.

But teens who have a vibrant relationship with their God then turn away from it, in response to loss, anger, or hopelessness, for instance, often fall into depression. Philosophers and scholars call this a "spiritual depression." The teenager recognizes that something important is spurned and is now lost to them. As with other losses, their failure to grieve, or to renew this spiritual relationship, causes them pain. As a physician caring for the entire patient, I must be sensitive to a patient's perceptions of the world in which they live, how they view the workings of that world, how this creates their own type of religion, and how this all makes sense in their relationship with God. Then, I must be able to help repair those losses if I can. Often, I'll suggest that teens get counseling not just from psychologists, but also from family and religious leaders.

Many teens describe sex as being spiritual. I agree with them. Sex is sacred and something extraordinary, during which a connection occurs beyond human comprehension. If they believe this is true, then sex indeed is something to be protected and cherished because it affects the spiritual dimension of their lives. Thus, when sex goes awry (or causes pain), that pain affects their spiritual life.

UNCOVERING DEPRESSION IN TEENS

Many healthy, normal teens will experience one or more episodes of brief depression during their adolescence. This happens for a number of reasons, including hormonal fluctuations, major life changes, and small and large losses. Understanding what happens during adolescence (as described in Chapter 10) will help you recognize normal changes in your teens as they occur, and become aware when something is really wrong. For while healthy, emotional upheaval in a teen can mimic depression, there are some major differences you should be on the lookout for.

Age-inappropriate behavior. It's normal for teenagers to act their appropriate age one day, then act years younger the next, then swerve back again. But when a teenager's behavior regresses and stays regressed for two or more weeks, there's cause for concern. For instance, a teen who normally likes going out in the evenings with friends, but stops, instead heading to bed early, may be depressed. Sometimes, depressed teens may even ask to sleep with their parents, particularly if they are experiencing anxiety. This is particularly common in girls who have been sexually assaulted or raped. They're seeking safety, but they're also exhibiting regressive behavior.

Emotional outbursts. As teenagers' hormones fluctuate wildly, it's normal to see occasional emotional outbursts and temper tantrums. These episodes may last a few days, then suddenly disappear. But depressed teens become angrier and angrier, and show more frequent outbursts that don't go away. They consistently erupt over small things, becoming irrationally angry and viewing the world only in black and white terms. For instance, while a healthy teen might argue with a sibling over sharing clothes, fighting only for a few minutes, a depressed teen might start crying, screaming, and even flailing her arms and legs. She might devise a scheme to retaliate later on and physically hurt her sibling, clearly displaying anger disproportionate to the conflict.

Sinking self-esteem. It's normal for a teenager's self-esteem to drop in early adolescence as they leave behind what they know (childish ways of thinking and acting) and venture into new, unknown areas. They want to behave like grown-ups and think like older teens, but they don't have a clue how to do that. So they feel insecure because they don't know who they are or where they're headed. But as maturity sets in and teens recognize new strengths, they begin liking themselves again and their self-esteem rises. Depressed teens, on the other hand, never like who they are. They see themselves through the dark glasses of depression, and feel negative about everything they think, feel, and do—most particularly, about themselves.

Frequent shifts in friends. Normally, teenagers expand their circle of friends and are part of one, two, or three groups. Although they may leave some friendships behind, they typically carry a few good ones forward while making new friends who have different interests and qualities. But when teens are depressed, they often completely cut their ties with old friends while forging relationships with kids they'd never have been interested in a few months earlier. This sudden transition to completely new friends is a sign of trouble.

Everyday changes. Other warning signs for depression include changes in eating patterns (lack of interest in food, or constant eating), changes in sleep patterns (never sleeping or sleeping all the time), and consistent changes in clothing and grooming styles, including tattooing and body piercing.

Actually, one of the best ways to determine whether your teenager is depressed is to simply ask. Kids who are really hurting, those who feel engulfed in a black cloud, yet who have a decent relationship with you, will tell you how they're feeling.

Like the cute 17-year-old who came into my office recently for a checkup and cheerfully chattered on about her involvement in sports, choir, and a host of other activities. When I asked if she felt happy about life in general, however, she burst into tears.

For the next ten minutes, she sobbed out the fact that for the past several months she'd been worried that she might be seriously depressed. She'd seen an advertisement on television for an antidepressant medication, she said, and when the announcer read out the symptoms of depression, she realized she experienced every one. We talked for a while and she was clearly relieved by our conversation. As it turned out, she'd been experiencing a mild form of depression that didn't require medication. Simply talking it out was enough.

This is common in teenagers. I've found that teens love talking about themselves and their feelings if they genuinely believe that you can offer them some relief.

So, if you're ever worried that something is wrong with your son or daughter, *start by asking*. You'll be amazed. They may just start talking. And that's when you need to listen.

PART II

The Forces at Work

SIX

■ Between 15 and 20% of young men and women have become infected with herpes by the time they reach adulthood.

Birth Control Is *Not* Disease Control

WITH MANY LANDMARK SCIENTIFIC advances comes a curse. Today we can clone human tissues but agonize over the ethics of doing so. We can save premature infants who weigh only a few ounces but struggle to find the funds to keep them alive. We can extend the lives of cancer patients with bone-marrow transplants and high-dose chemotherapy, but exhaust them and cause them great pain in the process.

When birth control pills arrived in the 1960s, our generation felt we had just what we needed to take ultimate charge of our sexual lives and our decisions about reproduction. But what we failed to see was the curse that accompanied it. "The pill" opened the way for sexual freedom and control, allowing sexual expression to reach new heights. It offered the ultimate "protection" to women who wanted to be sexually active. And it promised "safe sex." Only now are we coming to realize that safe sex isn't safe. In fact, it can be deadly.

How did we get lulled into this false sense of security? In our tunnel-vision mentality, the pill helped us to stay focused on only one consequence of sex: pregnancy. We obsessed about teen pregnancy. We watched news programs bemoan the plight of unwed mothers, and high-ranking government officials vow to do something about the national crisis of teen pregnancy. And birth control medications have successfully done just that. Teen pregnancy numbers *are* down.[1] What we didn't see was the growing numbers of sexually transmitted diseases. We are now cursed with escalating STD rates that have risen much faster than teen pregnancies have fallen. Many of us in medicine, education, and public health have made a terrible mistake as we diligently worked to keep our teens from having babies. We did such a good job promoting birth control, we have actually encouraged our kids to have sex younger, more often, and with more partners.

By telling our kids that contraception equals "safe sex," we have perpetrated a dangerous lie. The fact is, birth control *is not* disease control. And so, as easy-access contraception has become commonplace, the rates of teen sex have exploded, and the STD epidemic is in full force.

The realization that our society's overwhelming embrace of birth control has actually helped *cause* an epidemic of disease was difficult for me to accept—as both a doctor and a woman. Let me share with you my own story of conversion.

MY STORY

In 1987, I left Children's Hospital of Wisconsin behind me. I cried for days because I had loved working there so much. It was a strange mix of exhaustion, intense training, and grueling schedules that, while tough, was one of the most rewarding experiences of my life.

Ninety-hour workweeks for three straight years. I had sweated, bled (literally), and broken down when a patient died. My long white coat was stained from body fluids spilled from spinal taps, intubation procedures, and babies' tears. A part of me stayed in those halls; that's where I'd lost much of my innocence and grown up as a doctor—and as a person.

By that fall, however, I was ready to enter private practice. I was trained and I felt smart. My instructors had been some of the best in the country. I was ready to take on any medical problem thrown my way. And I believed I could make a difference in the lives of my new patients, particularly teenage girls.

I was tired of seeing teen girls giving birth to babies in our large inner-city clinic, and when I moved to the cushiness of private practice I was determined to change the future for any teen girl who fell in my path. What were my weapons?

The best and most powerful were a variety of oral contraceptives. These pills would help teen girls ward off pregnancy. Pregnancy meant babies, and babies shouldn't belong in their lives yet. Babies meant welfare, poverty, and minimal education.

My second weapon was words. I could talk to teens. Teens were— and still are—my passion. I would spend time reasoning with them that having babies was not in their best interest. I could help them, *get them to understand* that they shouldn't get pregnant. I wanted them to avoid pregnancy so badly that I joked with my colleagues about putting estrogen and progesterone in the city water. The sad part is, I was half serious.

Finally, I had my feminist ideals. I wanted to teach these young girls to like being young women, to not let boys trap them into sex, and to make sure they held themselves in high regard. I wanted they themselves, not boys, to make their sexual decisions. I wanted them to be in charge of their bodies. I wanted them to know that their bodies were important.

I also had the medical community at large behind me. We doctors, teachers, and public health officials would *do something* about teen pregnancy because it was a national crisis. Hundreds of thousands of teen girls were pregnant. Schools were wondering what to do with these young mothers-to-be. Abortion? Keep them in school? Send them home until after the baby's born? And what to do with the babies? Adoption? Social workers went crazy intervening for kids, adoption agencies grew, and the word "abortion" started fights in drugstores, supermarkets, and courtrooms across the country.

So I, like many of my colleagues, worked harder to prevent arguments and babies: Get the girls on birth control.

Personally, I waged war for about ten years with oral contraceptives in one pocket and (later on) an injection of Depo-Provera (an injectable hormone-based contraceptive) ready to go in the other.

I remember one young girl of about 15, who literally ran into my office one day without an appointment, pleading to be seen. She was 33 weeks pregnant and poor. She had just come from an appointment with her obstetrician, who wanted to perform an abortion on her. Why? Because he too was doing what he believed was the best way to curb unwanted teen births. While I found his method personally repulsive, I had to realize that he was impassioned to keep teens off the streets and in school. He, like me, wanted to keep our mutual patient free from the pains associated with being a teen parent. He simply used a different method than I did.

I was furious. *If he cared so much, why hadn't he gotten her on birth control pills so she wouldn't find herself in this dilemma? Why had he tried to coerce this young girl into doing something she didn't want? She deserved to make her own decisions!*

The girl was frightened and confused. She refused to have an abortion, even after he pushed her.

At the time, I helped her make some decisions. She would have the baby and focus on getting good care for it, and she would get it listed with a great adoption center. She did these things, and she eventually finished high school, during which time she found yet another boyfriend. This time, I was ready with my weapon. I made sure that she didn't repeat her "mistake." Every three months I pulled out the syringe-gun and shot her up with Depo-Provera. I helped her make sure she wouldn't get pregnant again. Until she was 19 and left my practice, she held pregnancy at bay.

Some four years later I ran into her again. My colleague told me he had just admitted a new patient to the hospital . . . she had mentioned my name. Did I know her? Had she been my pediatric patient? I acknowledged that she had. "What's wrong with her? What's she in for?" I asked.

"She presented to the ER with abdominal pain," he explained. "We ran a bunch of labs, worried she might have an ectopic pregnancy. She didn't. She has bad PID—probably Fitz-Hugh and Curtis syndrome. We're doing some liver functions, probably an MRI. I'll keep you posted, if you'd like. So sad—know what I mean? She's only 24."

Whammo. I felt sick. What had I done? My years of coaching her not to get pregnant had worked. But had I failed her? Now, at the age of 24, she lay in a hospital bed because of an STD. Probably gonorrhea or chlamydia. It had been in her body who knows how long, and now it was having a field day in her abdomen. The bacteria, perhaps even both types, had climbed up into her uterus and multiplied beyond it into her other internal organs. She had a raging infection, with pus in her abdominal cavity and around her liver and diaphragm. When she breathed, sharp pains shot into her right shoulder because a large nerve was involved. Now it was causing her liver problems, perhaps the infection was in her bloodstream. Certainly her fertility was in jeopardy—and maybe even her life.

I thought about the day she came into my office when she was 15. I was so blind and naïve, feeling that I was serving her better than her obstetrician, who wanted to perform an abortion. I felt proud that I could *really help*. Keep the mistake away. But here she lay, fighting for her life because no one—including me—saw what was coming. I didn't see the diseases like gonorrhea and chlamydia and all the rest waiting in the wings to explode in her young body and in millions of girls and boys like her around the country. I was as cruel to her as her obstetrician. Both of us failed to see what the real problem was. It wasn't pregnancy. It was the unrestricted sex that brought about the ravages of PID on this poor girl.

And it's the unrestricted sex that has brought about the onslaught of this epidemic.

I'm glad to say that my young patient didn't die from PID. But she is infertile and at 24 now faces her future unable to ever bear children.

THE SUCCESS OF BIRTH CONTROL

For the past 25 years or so, doctors like myself, public health officials, educators, and parents have been somewhat successful at reducing teen pregnancy and teen motherhood.

In 1980, for instance, the pregnancy rate for 15- to 17-year-old girls was approximately 75 per 1000 teens. As we health professionals saw this rate slowly rise during the 1980s until teen pregnancy hit a peak of 80 per 1000 in 1990, we aggressively campaigned to do something about it. We determined to push contraception—any contraception we felt teens would use. And we were successful. Over the 1990s, we saw the teen pregnancy rates slowly decline. In 1990, 80 teens out of 1000 became pregnant, but by 1997 that number had dropped to 63 per 1000.[2] This indeed has been a success.

The numbers for older teens, however, have been less impressive. Rates for teens 18 to 19 years old have fallen, but less dramatically. In 1980, for instance, the pregnancy rate was approximately 160 per 1000. It stayed fairly steady until it rose slightly during the early 1990s, then began to fall. By 1997, it was at its lowest in 17 years, at 140 per 1000 teens. Still, it is interesting to note how much higher the pregnancy rate for 18- to 19-year-old girls is than it is for 15- to 17-year-old girls. Just about twice as many 18- to 19-year-old girls get pregnant as 15- to 17-year-olds.[3]

Sexual activity among teens has skyrocketed since the 1950s, but pregnancy rates have declined. Clearly, the explosion in the use of contraceptives has "worked."

The success of falling teen pregnancy rates has been attributed to increased contraception use—in particular condoms and injectable and implanted contraception in girls—according to the National Vital Statistics Report.[4]

Now let's look at trends in contraception use in teens. In 1982, less than half of girls 15 to 19 years old used any form of contraception—including the pill or condoms—during their first act of sex. By 1995, three-fourths of the same population said they had used contraception at first intercourse.[5] Again, this shows our successes with public health efforts among our teens. Or does it ? Let's combine all of these numbers and trends and see where we are.

We know that since the sexual revolution took root in the 1970s, sexual freedom and sexual activity among our youth have risen dramatically. We not only see more teens sexually active, but we have seen younger and younger teens—some as young as 11 years old—start having sex.[6] Teen pregnancy began to rise and over the past two decades we beefed up efforts to curb the fallout of teen sex: pregnancy. And as we have seen, we have been successful. We have witnessed the swell of contraceptive use among teens including condoms, oral contraceptives ("the pill"), and injectable and implant contraceptives.

But in the midst of our "successes," what has happened over that same time period to STDs among our teens? They have exploded into epidemic proportions. While we physicians handed out oral contraceptives, chlamydia rates rose. While we gave injections of Depo-Provera, the numbers of HPV rose. And while we handed out condoms to teens, we saw syphilis outbreaks and genital herpes climb.

TOOLS FOR PROTECTION

So just what is this medical smorgasbord of birth control? Here's what doctors, educators, and other health officials have been pushing on our teens:

Oral contraceptives. We have a wide variety of oral contraceptives available to women in this country. And they're just as available to teens. Any teen can walk into Planned Parenthood and get birth control pills—often for free. They can go to their local general practitioner, family doctor, or pediatrician, make an appointment, and get them. Often they'll walk out of the doctor's office that same day with a handful of sample packs, to tide them over until they get the prescription filled. And most kids will have very few questions asked of them. Why? Because physicians and other health care providers are doing the best they can to halt teen pregnancy. And the truth is, oral contraceptives work extremely well in preventing pregnancy.

But one problem with teen girls being on the pill is that they don't always take the pills as they should. For the best protection against pregnancy, the pill should be taken at the same time every day. In my experience (and that of many of my colleagues), girls will start on birth control pills and then soon forget to take them. They'll forget to take a pill one day, then another day. Sometimes they take two in one day, then skip a few days. And many teen girls hesitate to take oral contraceptives because they fear gaining weight. (Some girls will gain a couple of pounds, many others do not.)

How many teen girls are currently taking oral contraceptives? It's hard to nail down exact numbers because many girls start, then stop right away. Still others get prescriptions in the privacy of their physician's office unbeknownst to parents or others. But research shows that 52% of 15- to 19-year-old girls have taken the pill, 9.8% have tried injectables (Depo-Provera), and 2.8% have tried implants (Norplant).[7] How soon are they taking them? *Some start taking the pill as soon as they begin to menstruate. For some girls, this can be as young as 13 or 14!*

Condoms. Condoms continue to be the contraception of choice for most teens.[8] They are quick and easy and don't need to be taken every day like birth control pills. And you don't need a prescription—you can simply buy them at the local drugstore or convenience store. Health officials boast that condom use among adolescents has dramatically increased, mainly because of the large campaigns by agencies to get kids using them. But as we'll see in the following chapters, condoms won't serve our teens well, because they offer inadequate protection from most STDs.

Long-term hormonal therapies. With the advent of Norplant and Depo-Provera, two distinct forms of long-term hormonal therapy, teens discovered that contraception could be quite easy. Health care workers recognized another important factor: These methods made it easy for teens to practice birth control. Norplant is inserted surgically beneath the skin of a girl's upper arm in the form of six thin, flexible plastic implants containing the hormone levonorgestrel. After this one-time insertion, Norplant can remain effective in preventing pregnancy for *5 years*. Imagine the freedom a teen girl would feel after it is in place, no longer having to worry, regardless of how often she has sex or how many partners she chooses.

Depo-Provera requires an injection every three months and it, too, offers girls great freedom from worry about pregnancy. In fact, in my experience, Depo-Provera is much more popular among teens than oral contraceptives, simply because they don't have to worry about taking a pill every day. And, like Norplant and oral contraceptives, Depo-Provera works well to prevent pregnancy if administered correctly.

But, like most other forms of birth control, there is one major problem with the use of these long-term contraceptives: Teens are still completely vulnerable to every viral and bacterial STD possible. Even the minor protection that condoms afford is gone, because teens are less likely to use condoms when using long-term contraceptives.[9]

Other options. Other forms of contraception are available to teens, both by prescription or over the counter, but these are much less popular because they can have serious side effects or they may be cumbersome to use. The over-the-counter methods available include spermicides and female condoms. Other methods, for which a girl must be fitted or given a prescription, are the IUD, the diaphragm, and the cervical cap. But here again, the main focus of these methods is birth control, not disease prevention. I had one mother ask me to fit her 11-year-old daughter for an IUD! (I refused, of course.)

THE DOCTORS' DILEMMA

Only now has the magnitude and reality of the STD epidemic hit birth control advocates squarely in the face. And all of this creates a serious dilemma for doctors like myself.

Twenty years ago, I wouldn't have hesitated to prescribe oral contraceptives to teenage girls. In fact, *any* form of birth control was fine with me, as long as the patient used it consistently. As a young doctor swept away by the message of "safe" sex, I didn't know any better. To me, "safe" meant not getting pregnant. I was so focused on the pregnancy epidemic that I wrote hundreds of prescriptions for birth control pills and gave more injections of Depo-Provera than I care to remember.

But today, I think long and hard about prescribing birth control pills or Depo-Provera to kids because this puts them in such grave danger of contracting an STD. In giving a girl birth control that I know will protect her from pregnancy, am I inadvertently encouraging her to pick up a sexually transmitted disease?

And if you might ask, "What about condoms?" read on. We place far too much trust in those slim packets of latex and lambskin. In most cases, the chances of condoms preventing STDs is almost as thin as the condoms themselves. Hence, I think carefully about advising teens to use condoms, as well as other forms of birth control. The risks are just too high.

SEVEN

■ An NIH report on condom effectiveness revealed that condoms help reduce the risk of HIV transmission but fare poorly against other infections, particularly those transmitted via skin-to-skin contact—such as HPV and herpes.

Condoms and the Myth of Safe Sex

WHERE SEXUAL HEALTH IS CONCERNED, the nation is full of condom mania. Even as parents and educators wring their hands over adolescent pregnancy and STDs, many grin with relief and hold up a slim foil packet as the "solution." (I see this at every conference I attend.) An estimated 400 high schools in the United States make condoms available to students.[1] And many kids are using them.

Indeed, condom use by adolescents has skyrocketed during the past 20 years. Condom use among teens has increased from about 21% among sexually active boys ages 17 to 19 to nearly 67% in 1995.[2] Other data from 1997 shows that about half of adolescent girls in grades nine through twelve said they used a condom during their last sexual intercourse, compared with just over one-third in 1991.[3]

In a way, we might view all this as a victory. After all, there has been a slight drop in the number of teenage pregnancies.

But the problem is this: *During that same time period, the number of cases of kids with STDs has grown to epidemic proportions.*

Condoms, the only form of birth control purported to stop disease and the spread of STDs, *don't work.* "Safe" sex isn't safe. And the epidemic of STDs is due in part to this overconfident reliance on condoms.

To start at the beginning, we have to untangle a snarled web of misinformation, and we have to see this through the eyes and lifestyles of our kids. Consider Karen.

Karen's Story

Karen was one of those kids who drive you absolutely crazy. The way she could defy logic and self-righteously twist the facts of any situation to suit her own fancy would tie me in knots and leave me speechless after five minutes of conversation. She was one of the few patients I've ever had whom I secretly wanted to spank. Now, I'm not a spanker, but kids like Karen make me understand the rationale for it. Yet she was sweet, lively, optimistic, fun, endearing—and totally exasperating. I couldn't help but love her.

When Karen turned 17, she lost her bossy tone, and she stopped snarling at me like I was a dummy whenever I gave her hard, straightforward advice. When I saw her for a physical that year, we began talking about what was going on in her life, about family, friends, pompom tryouts—and Aaron, the latest love in her life. He was a senior, she was a junior. She described him as the "perfect guy." He was tall, had dark hair and eyes, and was "exciting to be with."

Exciting to be with? All my red flags went up. I knew from my experience with so many teenagers that "exciting" was not the same as "fun." Fun meant laughter and companionship. Exciting was something different altogether.

She continued giddily, "Oh, he's gorgeous. And he's not like any other guy I've been with. He lives on the edge, know what I mean? He likes being baaad."

Now my red flags were putting up red flags. "Bad" was often a code word for "in trouble with the law." I had a sense of dread about Aaron, but I tried not to let her know it.

"I got a picture, wanna see?" She jumped off my exam table, grabbed her purse, rifled through it, and produced a snapshot. I sighed. Aaron had a dog collar around his neck, complete with studs, three silver hoops in one ear, and a bar through his lip. But there was something else. His eyes weren't smiling. And they weren't sad. They were glaring at the camera, like he was ready to hit the person taking the photo. Aaron looked angry, and mean.

She watched me study the picture, reading my face and my body language. She wanted a positive response from me to make her feel better—maybe just a word that would let her know I approved of Aaron, that I thought he looked perfect too. I tried to hide my worry. I failed.

"You think just like my parents do," she said, sounding disappointed. "They don't like him either."

I've seen girls and boys react in this way before. Searching for excitement, they seek out a girlfriend or boyfriend who can lead them into dangerous places, both physically and emotionally. As often as not, this meant becoming sexually active, and Karen had dropped plenty of hints during our conversation that sex was exactly the kind of excitement she meant. As we finished up her physical, I asked her about it.

"So Karen, tell me about sex with Aaron. What's up?" I said.

"Oh, I don't know. We do have sex, Dr. Meeker, and I know how you feel about that. I know you've told me it can be dangerous. But, you need to know that we *always* use protection. That's one of the really good things about Aaron. He's responsible and he really watches out for me."

"Do you guys have sex a lot?"

"Yeah. I guess so. Couple times a week. You know, when I told you about the condom thing, I know he does it 'cause he respects me. He really doesn't like them. He always starts without one, then puts one on when we're almost done. That's what I mean. He stops right in the middle. A lot of guys wouldn't use one at all."

I sighed. I was tired of untangling misinformation about condoms from the truth, and I was tired of being angry that she and other kids like her had been led to believe that condoms would keep them safe from STDs and pregnancy. I took a deep breath and told her the facts.

"Karen, one of the things that I love about you is your honesty. You are maturing and I'm so proud to see you thinking and trying to act responsibly. But I need to talk with you about condoms and about you and Aaron. Two problems. First, condoms do you no good if he doesn't use it until halfway through. He can leak semen before putting it on, which could make you pregnant, or if he has an infection, make you sick. Here's the other part. Some germs—some pretty bad ones—spread from areas of his skin that *aren't* covered by a condom. I sure wish this were simpler, but it isn't. The bottom line is, there's *always* a risk with sex. A risk of getting pregnant or a risk of getting an infection, or even both. And some of those infections can cause cancer or problems with you being able to have babies when you're older. What are your thoughts about that?"

I could only hope she had taken the information I had offered seriously, but she became instantly defensive.

"Oh, I don't know. He's just so much fun. And I guess part of me knew that maybe we weren't real safe. But cancer? No way. Look, Dr. Meeker, I know Aaron doesn't have any, you know, diseases. He'd tell me for sure."

Somehow I wasn't as convinced about that as Karen was.

"Karen, you could be right. Maybe he doesn't have any diseases. The problem is, most of the ones he might have usually don't give guys symptoms. Besides," I said, "have you ever looked to see if he's got anything?"

"Oh, Dr. Meeker, come on, you've got to be kidding. I wouldn't do *that*!" Her embarrassment was obvious.

By the time our appointment ended, despite all my efforts to get through to Karen, I knew I hadn't been successful.

Several years went by, during which she broke up with Aaron and dated several more boys. Condoms made her feel "protected," she said at a later visit, so she saw no reason to give up sex. But she became a little complacent—after all, none of my dire predictions had come true—and eventually became careless about "protection."

In her early 20s, however, that beautiful, Gap-clad girl who smelled like springtime contracted HIV. Like many girls her age, she had been insisting on condom use *sometimes*. But not *always*. It's one of the problems with condoms: To gain any protection from disease, you need to use them *every time* you have sex. No misses. You must be perfect. But can anyone be?

Karen hasn't developed AIDS yet. There's not much she can do but wait and try to live as normal a life as she can. She finished college and has a good job, but she doesn't know from day to day when signs of the fatal strike of AIDS will come.

TALKING TERMS

So why aren't condoms doing the job they're supposed to do? Why aren't they protecting the Karens of the world? You need to know, for the sake of your own teens, the difference between fact and hype where condoms are concerned. Unfortunately, that means repeating some bad news: *Condoms are no solution*.

I can hear your objections already: "No solution? What about 'safe sex'"?

During the 1990s, these two words became the mantra of health educators in schools and health care clinics for teens across the country, and code words for using condoms. But how do we know that condoms are safe? And what does "safe" mean? We must be clear about definitions, because I'm a stickler for making sure that both teens and parents understand the risks.

The term "safe" means that a person won't get harmed or sick. And so does the word "protected." So when we tell teens that the way to have "safe sex" is to use condoms, which are perceived as "protection," we're implying that they'll be protected from harm and disease. So that's what they hear: If they use condoms, nothing bad like STDs or pregnancy will happen to them.

Medically, however, this just isn't true. The best that condoms can do is *reduce* a person's risk for contracting disease. Even if condoms are used perfectly, 100% of the time, risk still exists. That risk is that the condom will slip or break about 2 to 4% of the time.[4] And that's just the beginning. We also have to factor in what disease the condom is supposed to prevent. Gonorrhea? Syphilis? HPV? HIV? The risk of getting any one of these differs with a condom. The truth is, condoms do best in reducing the risk of HIV, but they're much worse with many other STDs (we'll look at these in a moment). The levels of safety are much lower than you think.

I have a problem with the word "safe." It makes kids feel that they won't get pregnant or catch a disease if they use condoms. But it's not true. We need to tell kids that reducing the risks is not the same as being safe. We need to tell them exactly what the risks are, and what condoms can and cannot do. We must be honest with our kids. It could save their lives.

THE REAL DEAL ON CONDOMS

How much do condoms really reduce the risk of our kids becoming infected with disease? Our best information comes from a panel of 28 medical experts in a recent report sponsored by the National Institutes of Health. The group comprised men and women, practicing physicians and researchers, liberals and conservatives, all trained to have their fingers on the pulse of the spread and prevention of STDs in the United States. They gathered for a two-day workshop in Herndon, Virginia, in June 2000, to evaluate the effectiveness of condoms. Thirteen months later they released their findings

They concluded that, while latex condoms could reduce the transmission of HIV/AIDS and gonorrhea in males, there was *not enough evidence to determine that they were effective in reducing the risk of most other sexually transmitted diseases.*[5]

The report unleashed a firestorm of reaction, with numerous physicians' groups and members of Congress calling for the immediate resignation of then-CDC director Dr. Jeffrey Koplan, for hiding and misrepresenting vital medical information that showed condoms don't fully protect against STD transmission. "The failure of public health efforts to prevent the STD epidemic in America is related to the CDC's 'safe-sex' promotion and its attempts to withhold from the American people the truth of condom ineffectiveness," group members said.[6]

Unfortunately, this firestorm quickly died down. Today if you ask most adults (or teens) about the best way to prevent STDs, they will answer with one smug word: condoms.

They're wrong.

SEX, LIES, AND THE FREEDOM OF INFORMATION ACT

It should come as no surprise that when the NIH report was completed, some health officials considered keeping it private. The shocking findings in the report contradicted nearly a decade of official government reproductive health policy. As the *Washington Post* reported in July 2001, it was only after pressure from some conservative organizations and the threat of a Freedom of Information Act request that the report was released to the public.[7]

Overall, if used *correctly* and *consistently*, condoms rarely fail to prevent the passage of a virus or bacteria in bodily fluid. That's good. The problem is, not all STDs are transmitted through fluid. We saw in the last chapter that although *some* STDs are spread through sexual fluids, such as semen and vaginal fluids, others, including HPV and herpes, are transmitted from one person to another through skin contact. Also, certain concentrations of viruses and bacteria are required for infections to occur, sometimes very small, depending on which bug you're dealing with. Specifically, here's what the panel found:

Condoms may help somewhat. When used 100% of the time, condoms can reduce the risk of sexually transmitted HIV infections in both sexes and the risk of gonorrhea in men by about 85%.[8] Now, an 85% protection rate may sound good, but it's not good enough for my patients, their parents, or me. My job is to keep my patients disease-free. I didn't take the Hippocratic Oath to make sure they remained disease-free 85% of the time. I took it to keep them healthy 100% of the time.

And remember, 85% risk reduction represents the *very best possible scenario*. That means that if a condom is used every time a person has intercourse, and is used correctly all of the time, then there is an 85% chance that he or she won't get HIV or gonorrhea. Now, if this were your teen putting on a condom, would 85% be good enough? He still has a 15% chance that he will get HIV. That doesn't sound like "protection" or "safe sex" to me.

Sometimes condoms don't help at all. The best medical literature available to us on condoms also shows that only "insufficient evidence" exists with regard to their effectiveness in preventing other STDs.[9] Research currently under way will help us better understand the real track record of condoms over time. Until we get more answers, it would be easy to tell our teens just to use condoms to be on the safe side, but the situation is not that simple, and such advice would be grossly misleading.

First, every STD has its own characteristics, its individual personality. Gonorrhea behaves differently from chlamydia, which behaves differently from herpes and HIV. Some STDs are viruses, some are bacteria. Some live on skin, some in blood, some only in genital fluids. The amount of germs needed to cause an infection varies from one disease to another.

Ways of transmitting the disease also vary. Some sexual practices put certain parts of the body in contact with other parts of a partner's body. (I'll talk about this in greater detail in Chapter 9.) But condoms don't protect against *all* forms of disease transmission. Condoms only prevent contact with *some* bodily fluids and *only* the skin of the genitals themselves.

Second, for us to really determine whether condoms protect our kids, we need to know if teens wear them all the time and if they wear them correctly. If a teen wears a condom only half the time, how well is he protected? *Not at all*. Or if he puts it on the wrong way, how much disease risk reduction does he get? *Not much*.

So a statement like, "The use of condoms in teens has skyrocketed over the past 20 years" might make us feel better if we accept it at face value. But are those teens using them like Aaron did? Are they wearing them *every time* they have intercourse? Do they know how to put them on correctly?

See how tough this gets? You need to know the real risk your kids take when they say they are using condoms, so you can help them make informed decisions.

Finally, many teens engage in higher-risk sexual activity than do most adults. They have multiple partners, they have anal sex, oral sex, and group sex in addition to traditional vaginal-penile inter-course. If a boy is engaging in group sex, does he change his condom every time he changes partners so he doesn't carry germs from one person to another? If he's receiving oral sex, does he ever bother to wear a condom? You begin to see the scope of the problem.

CONDOMS VERSUS THE STDS

If we want to make sound judgments and give good advice to our teens, we need to review the best available literature done on sex and the effectiveness of condoms in the context of all of these variables and complications.

But we're not completely in the dark. Here's what the best medical literature available on condoms tells us about condoms and specific diseases.

Gonorrhea. The NIH panel found six studies—four of men and two of women—on gonorrhea and condom effectiveness that were "acceptable for review." That means the studies were rigorously controlled so that the data they provide is believable and accurate, and demonstrates what the researchers say they demonstrate. Although the studies led the panel to conclude that condoms can reduce a man's risk of contracting gonorrhea, the studies weren't as clear for women.[10] Recently, however, newer data has come from a study in Uganda, where HIV and gonorrhea are at a crisis level. That country has implemented aggressive campaigns to reduce the spread of both diseases. In their research, they are finding that any person who *always* wears a condom during sex reduces his or her risk of getting gonorrhea by about 50%.[11] So even if you use condoms in the most "responsible" way imaginable, you're still playing with fire when it comes to gonorrhea. Again, think of your own kids. Does a one in two chance sound like good odds to you?

HPV. Volumes of good medical research are appearing on HPV because it has erupted onto the medical scene so furiously. HPV, more than any of the STDs, has dealt the death blow to condoms. Let me tell you why. Physicians and researchers came to grips a couple of years ago with the fact that HPV was spreading like wildfire and condoms fared poorly, at best, in helping to prevent its spread. The latest studies report that "condoms have *no impact* on the risk of sexual transmission of human papilloma virus in women."[12] And there is no clear evidence that condoms reduced HPV transmission in men.[13] Condoms offer inadequate protection against HPV because it is highly contagious, and it's spread by skin-to-skin contact as well as through secretions. So latex condoms may fail to prevent transmission of HPV in women because the virus may be present on areas of skin not covered by the condom. The bottom line is that we cannot tell our kids that they are protected from HPV and cervical cancer simply by using condoms.

Finally, we know that teen girls who repeatedly have sex and get exposed to cancer-producing strains of HPV are the ones who are at higher risk for cervical cancer. But giving a "safe sex" message about condoms to girls can make them feel, falsely, that they're adequately protected against HPV. Feeling so safe may actually encourage them to feel okay about having more and more sex in the future, thus further increasing their risk for exposure and possible cancer further down the road, perhaps even during their child-bearing years.

Herpes. One of the best studies on condoms and herpes was published in the *Journal of the American Medical Association* in June 2001. The study followed monogamous couples in which one partner had herpes and the other didn't. Even among these highly motivated people, only 60% ever used condoms, and a mere 13% used condoms consistently. Even among those who used condoms, however, the study found only the woman's risk of getting herpes was reduced. *Using condoms didn't help the men reduce their risk of getting the disease at all.*[14]

These findings don't surprise me. Remember that the herpes virus, like the HPV virus, is spread from skin to skin, not just genitals to genitals. Since a condom covers only the penis, an ulcer on the shaft or glans (head) of a boy's penis would be covered. But if a girl has an ulcer on her labia, it could easily touch an uncovered area of her partner's skin. And, of course, someone with the virus may be infectious, or shedding the virus, even if there are no visible lesions.

Chlamydia. The research on the effectiveness of condoms in preventing chlamydia is not encouraging. Two out of three studies in women found no protection from condoms. How well are men protected by condoms from chlamydia? Studies show that "they may or may not reduce the risk of chlamydia in men."[15] Overall, though, the panel concluded, "other studies in men and women demonstrated either no or some protection or are inconclusive." Since the NIH stated that "the evidence is inconclusive" about whether condoms do or do not work against chlamydia, subsequent data has appeared. The studies from Uganda show that when men "always" wore condoms, the effectiveness of condoms in reducing the risk of their partner getting infected was 50%.[16] While this study was done in men (some young adults, some older), it is important to try to find a "best-case scenario" so that we might extrapolate how well our teens might do.

In other words, if teens and adults, knowing that their use of condoms is being studied, have sex and reduce their partners' risk of getting chlamydia by 50%, we might fairly safely assume that condoms would help with about the same effectiveness, if they wear condoms every time they have sex.

Syphilis. Many studies exist on condoms and syphilis. What do they show? Studies on adults show that condoms can help reduce the risk of getting syphilis, but condoms must be worn all the time. This is the tricky part—particularly for teens. One study looking at how well condoms decreased the risk of getting syphilis was done on prostitutes (well trained in condom use and highly motivated). The study showed that among adults who always used condoms, the risk of getting syphilis went down by 30%.[17] But that also means that 70% were at a relative risk. Another study done in Uganda found similar results.[18]

Trichomoniasis. The lack of available studies meant that the NIH panel could reach no conclusion. While one limited study showed a small amount of protection from trichomonas for women who used condoms, the bottom line is that still there is no clear evidence that condoms afford women protection from trichomonas. And one study done since the NIH conference looking at people who "always" used condoms confirmed this.[19]

WHAT TEENS FEAR MOST

For decades we've been giving the same time-honored advice to young men who are coming of age: If you're going to have sex, at least use a condom. You'll hit a double-header—protection against unwanted pregnancies and defense against disease.

It was a powerful argument, and our boys listened. Teens themselves are more frightened of pregnancy than disease because, from their perspective, a baby will disrupt their lives more than an infection—particularly an infection that has no symptoms and may not cause harm until "years down the road."

As difficult as it can be to make a teen understand the consequences of sexual behaviors, it is easier to help them appreciate the reality of teen pregnancy than the reality of the STD epidemic. First, teens hear more about pregnancy. We have been on the bandwagon of curbing teen pregnancy longer than we've been trying to stop teen STDs. In short, teens are more aware because we've educated them.

Second, teens can't see infections, but they can see a swollen belly. They can see a girl at school growing large with pregnancy. Unfortunately, most times, teens who have an STD or two don't have symptoms. This doesn't help them or us because they live with infections they don't realize they have, and don't seek treatment.

Third, teens are often egocentric. Pregnancy puts them out. It can't be cured with a shot of antibiotic or a handful of pills. Babies force teens to make tough decisions. They require a total lifestyle change. Teens can grasp the reality of that. All of this makes teens respect pregnancy more—and fear it more—than STDs.

Finally, teens don't want to let their parents down or get them upset. Telling a parent that she has an infection is easier for many teens than telling a parent she's pregnant. Again, this relates to a fear. Fear of telling mom or dad motivates some teens to prevent pregnancy rather than STDs if any preventative measures are to be taken at all.

CONDOMS AND TEENAGERS: AN UNHEALTHY MIX

Of course, part of the problem with condoms lies with teenagers themselves. Here are some of the reasons why:

The longer a teenager stays in a relationship, the less likely he is to use condoms.[20] I see this all the time. There are lots of kids who stay in relatively long-term relationships with each other. (Long-term for you and me is maybe five years, for a teen it may be six to nine months.) They don't jump around from one boyfriend or girlfriend to another. While this form of monogamy is good, it also poses problems for me or any other doctor.

Michael's story is typical. He and Gwen started dating their sophomore year in high school. They fell in love and stayed committed to each other. They agreed not to date other people and from all I could see, they didn't. They enjoyed each other's company greatly. They studied together, talked endlessly on the phone (so Gwen's mother complained), and they frequently spent time at each other's home.

Early in their relationship I asked Michael about his sexual activity with Gwen. He said there was none; that he wanted to hold off. But as time went on and their love grew deeper, they started having sex. He told me then that he "always" used a condom because they didn't want Gwen to get pregnant. Interestingly, he shook his head when I asked him if he was afraid of infections.

"No way," he'd said. "Not with Gwen." She was probably a virgin when they began dating and I'm pretty sure Michael was. As time went on, however, he started getting "lazy" (his word) about using condoms. This made me crazy. I told him that pregnancy was very much a real risk and that using condoms "once in a while" was asking for trouble.

I had difficulty getting through to him for a couple of reasons. First, sex was still new territory to him, by and large. He hadn't done it long enough to really understand that he could get in trouble, and a sense of caution hadn't yet developed deep roots in him. Second, a part of him believed that Gwen would never get pregnant. And the longer they had sex without her getting pregnant, the more that kind of adolescent, magical thinking was reinforced.

As far as STDs are concerned, I have consistently seen teens relax in their condom use. After they have sex, gain familiarity with their partner, and see that they haven't gotten an STD, they figure it's not an issue. What they fail to realize is that their partner may be having sex with another infected person while they're dating, or that they may, in fact, have a symptomless STD and not know it.

The bottom line with teens is that familiarity breeds complacency, and when that happens, condom use falls by the wayside.

The earlier a young girl becomes sexually active, the more likely she is to have a greater number of partners and reduce her insistence on condom use.[21] This is a loaded issue. First, many teen girls start having sex for reasons other than sexual drive. Young teens who are 12, 13, or 14 often have sex because they want attention, they want to be held, they want a baby to love, or they want attention from a male who reminds them of their father. With this last motivation, we've seen thousands of young teen girls get pregnant by men over the age of 20.

Young girls may be preyed upon, too. I recently spoke with a 19-year-old girl who told me she was giving her 13-year-old sister tips about negotiating her way through her first year of high school. The two sisters live in a large Midwestern city and attend a local public school. The older girl advised her sister: "Stay away from the senior boys. They're known for going after the freshman girls because they know they'll get oral sex from them."

Many young girls have difficulty telling an older boy to stay away sexually. They haven't yet learned assertiveness skills and are shy and hesitant. Plus, many young girls feel good when an older guy shows them attention. (Ever heard a mother boast about her sophomore daughter going to prom with the captain of the football team? I have.) Young girls can't handle older guys socially—they're not ready.

Many girls have more partners because they become desensitized to sex early on. I've talked with dozens of girls who've had four or more partners by the age of 16. When I ask if they really enjoy having sex, they shrug their shoulders. Then, if I ask them why they're having it, those same girls almost always say, "Why not? I've done it so many times, what's a few more?"

I've also found that when a girl gives away her virginity too early, it's often because she feels there is nothing about herself that's precious enough to protect. Many end up feeling used, and their self-image becomes even worse. I know this because they tell me. And I can see it in their body language.

As much as some adults may say that sex isn't something special ("it's just another healthy teen activity"), I've seen the faces and heard the voices of teens who know better. They know that it *is* special and that it *is* private. And when they let someone else share something that is so very private at too young an age, they get numb toward it. Eventually, their numbness may extend to carelessness about their health, so that condom use gets waved away.

I saw this happen to Chelsey. She first came to see me—or should I say, was forced to see me—at 15. She'd been vacationing with her family in a sunny resort in Mexico over spring break. During the week, she sneaked out at night to party with new-found friends, and had sex with a boy she met on the beach. Several weeks after she returned home, she missed her period. She told her mother. Later, her mother told her father. Her parents were horrified, and her mother dragged her into my office to find out if she was pregnant, and if she wasn't, to get her on birth control pills.

I did a pregnancy test and it came back negative. I gave her oral contraceptives for the time being and told her that I wanted to see her back soon.

After five visits, I learned that her beach episode was just one of many such encounters. In fact, she had her first sexual experience at 13 while in the eighth grade. At that age, she believed she was fat, a poor athlete and student, and had been worried about losing her friends. She met Jack that year. He was 16, cute, and very popular. She said that when he started paying attention to her, she felt good. If he liked her, she thought, then she must be "okay." "He made me feel good about myself," she said.

Three weeks after they started having sex, Jack dumped her. "That's when I really started to lose it," she remembered. She told me that she felt used, mad, and sad. She knew she had given something special to him, even though she hadn't thought about it at the time. She trusted him. She had been naked in front of him, and now, as she spoke about her relationship two years earlier, I could see that her painful feelings were still fresh. They were real and they were confusing.

Chelsey also came to realize that the Jack relationship set her up for more problems afterward. She said that after her breakup with Jack, she felt like a loser. So she decided to try to get another boyfriend. He wasn't as good-looking as Jack, but at the time she didn't care. She went out with him, they had sex, then broke up. After that relationship, Chelsey said that she "definitely" became numb to sex. "It was just something that I expected to do. I figured that all guys wanted it, so what the heck," she told me. The more sex she had, the more numb she became. She didn't like it, she didn't dislike it.

I asked about condoms. Did she ever use them? She shrugged her shoulders. "With Jack, sometimes. After that, I figured, why bother? If my boyfriend had 'em we'd use 'em, if not, it wasn't a big deal. I guess I was just lucky. I never really thought that I might get pregnant until the vacation in Mexico. I never got pregnant, don't think I got an infection, and after a while I just didn't seem to care."

That first day in my office, Chelsey's mother told me the girl needed birth control. In truth, Chelsey needed a lot more than birth control. She needed to break from her cycle of sex with boys. She needed help getting her self-esteem back, and she needed help learning to care about herself more.

Too few teenagers use condoms consistently or correctly.[22] Between 1993 and 1995, three studies examined the use of condoms among heterosexual couples in a committed relationship in which one partner was HIV-positive. Amazingly, these studies show that only about 50% of the couples always used condoms.[23] Now think about the meaning of this for a moment. The couples were mature and committed to each other. One of the partners had HIV and knew that if he or she didn't insist on condoms, the other parner's life would be at risk. Still, only half of the couples used condoms all of the time!

If adult, committed couples who were aware of the grave risks inherent in *not* using condoms were this inconsistent, we can reasonably assume (since all condom data on consistency of teen condom use is not yet in) that teens will use them even less consistently.

Less than half of adolescent boys (45%)[24] say they use condoms for every act of intercourse, and older teens (age 18 and 19) actually use condoms *less* than younger teens (age 15 to 17).[25] Remember, these are the same kids who forget to do their homework, brush their teeth, or take the dog out. Can we really expect them to use condoms each and every time they have sex?

Even if they start out using condoms in a relationship, after about three weeks, condom use falls. Perhaps teens feel (as adults do) that these "long-term" relationships are safer. Perhaps they trust their partner more.

Just as dangerous as inconsistent use of condoms is *incorrect* use. For a condom to work, it must be worn during the entire sexual encounter, be placed with the correct side out, and be held in place while the penis is withdrawn from the vagina. Yet one study found that one-third of male college students who used condoms consistently (very motivated if they always used them) were potentially exposed to an STD because their condoms slipped, broke, or were used incorrectly.[26]

In addition, the studies on male university students found that about one-third of them had accidentally tried to put their condoms on inside out at one time or another.[27] What happens is that a boy takes the condom out, puts it against his penis, and tries to unroll it. Then he realizes he has the wrong side exposed, turns it over, and puts it on the right way. This is called "flipping." Now let's suppose he had gonorrhea. He might have a drop of pus or seminal fluid at the end of his penis that would have touched the condom. When he flips it over, that drop of gonorrhea-infected fluid is on the outside of the condom, waiting to come up against his partner's vagina or cervix.

Overall, about one in three of the men surveyed wound up having unprotected intercourse either because they used the condom the wrong way or it broke. This is extremely important to understand. The study took male college students who were sexually experienced. They were clearly informed that they were in a study so that they would be especially careful about how they used their condoms. These men were intellectually and cognitively more mature than the teens we're talking about. The men clearly knew how to use condoms, yet look how much risk they still exposed their partners to.[28]

The problems aren't limited to college-age men. The National Longitudinal Study of Adolescent Health, the linchpin study of teenager health and behaviors, examined common misconceptions about correct condom use among 16,667 adolescents age 15 to 21, and found their answers to the following statements were wrong.

When putting on a condom, it is important to have it fit tightly, leaving no space at the tip. One-third of sexually active girls and two-thirds of boys who reported using condoms incorrectly identified this statement as true. It is false.

Vaseline can be used with condoms, and they will work just as well. Nearly one-third of sexually active girls (28%) and boys (34%) who'd used condoms incorrectly identified this statement as true. It is false.

Natural skin (lambskin) condoms provide better protection against the AIDS virus than latex condoms. Sixteen percent of girls and 25% of boys who'd used condoms during sex incorrectly identified this statement as true.[29]

The conclusion is inescapable: Even if condoms worked perfectly for every disease (which they don't), in the hands of a typically forgetful, impulsive, misinformed teenager, they are unlikely to be effective.

SENDING THE WRONG MESSAGE

News of the STD epidemic shocks us all. And once you understand that condoms don't keep our kids safe, the news can seem even more overwhelming. But we must deal with it head-on. Condoms have lulled us into complacency too long. They have provided a stopgap measure that can no longer hold back the flood of STDs. Our reliance on condoms has played a key role in the spread of disease, along with the major influences of the media and the new sexual habits of kids, as you'll see shortly.

EIGHT

■ The American Psychological Association estimates that teenagers are exposed to 14,000 sexual references and innuendoes a year on television alone.

Media and the World Our Kids See

SARAH IS A BEAUTIFUL 15-YEAR-OLD high school sophomore who chats feverishly and plays soccer like a pro. As I was giving her a physical exam in my office recently, I noticed she'd brought a magazine with her, probably because she's accustomed to waiting for me. It was *Cosmopolitan*. I asked her if it contained any worthwhile articles. She replied that she'd just bought it. She really hadn't read it yet. She glanced at the cover, giggled, and started reading titles: "Seven Bad-Girl Bedroom Moves You Must Master," "Erotic Tips to . . . " She stopped, blushing with embarrassment.

As I began examining her, Sarah changed the subject. She chatted excitedly about her new boyfriend, Brian, a 17-year-old she'd met at school. They often went to movies together, rented videos, and watched TV at each other's homes. They'd only been dating a couple of months and had decided to hold off from sex (they'd agreed neither was ready), which was good, because Sarah had already had sex with one other boyfriend and really hadn't enjoyed the experience. I verbally applauded her decision to wait and told her she was a mature young woman who was making excellent choices. But as we talked, my eyes kept drifting back to that magazine, which she had set down on a nearby chair. I wondered what effect those articles might exert on this young child's mind, and what I could possibly do to lessen that effect.

I get 45 minutes of an adolescent's time once every six months. Since a young girl is sexually active, and therefore at higher risk for diseases and pregnancy, I insist she see me that often. But the media gets hundreds of hours of her time. Beyond magazine articles, studies find American teenagers are exposed to an average of 38 hours a week of various media, including television, videos, music, computers, and video games. Everywhere I look, sex is used to sell stuff to our kids—whether it's blue jeans, perfume, or television shows. The American Psychological Association estimates that teenagers are exposed to 14,000 sexual references and innuendoes a year on television alone—all subtly (or not so subtly) influencing my patients into having sex, an act that can physically and mentally harm, if not kill them. That's scary, especially when you consider that young teens (ages 13 to 15) rank entertainment media as their top source of information about sexuality and sexual health.[1]

I often feel that the media and I are at war. They seduce Sarah to get sick; I try to keep her well.

Think I'm exaggerating? Check out the magazine covers at the supermarket next time you're there. Here's what Sarah and girls like her are reading:

"10 Dates before Sex? And Other Secrets of Love that Last and Last"

"Ultra Orgasms"

"Love Positions"

"Lust advice.com"

"Five Sex Moves Every Woman Must Know"

"20 Earth-Quaking Moves That Will Make Him Plead For Mercy And Beg For More"

"OH-OH Orgasms"

"New Bedroom Tricks To Try Tonight. Warning: Close The Windows"

" Play the Pick-up Game"

"Men Can't Resist Me"

"Eight Sex Pots Reveal Their Secret Weapons"

You get the picture. The gorgeous beauties gracing the covers were sexy, seductive, and staring right at the viewer. None wore visible wedding rings. One article included pictures of the different positions couples should try during intercourse. (Ironically, as I was researching this chapter, my own teenage daughter was helping, and yelled at me when she came across these depictions.) According to one study, 40% of female models in glossy magazines were considered "provocatively" dressed, up from 28% in 1983, and 18% of the men were in various states of undress, an increase from 11%.[2]

Then there are the advertisements. Seventeen percent of magazine ads containing at least one man and one woman depicted or implied intercourse in 1993, up from 1% ten years earlier.[3] You can bet the numbers are much higher today. Just the words are suggestive. A shampoo ad promised a totally "organic experience" if used, and a certain hair color boasted that its user "went all the way." But the words pale in comparison to the visual imagery. An ad for Versace eyeglasses depicts a bare-breasted woman standing in full frontal view behind a woman wearing the cool glasses. (I still don't remember what the glasses looked like, but I do still see those naked, tanned breasts.) Women modeling bathing suits sit with their legs splayed open in front of the camera.

When it comes to selling sex to our kids, Abercrombie & Fitch is one of the worst offenders. Their catalogue is filled with sexual content—complete with nudity and seductive positions. The company claims one must be over 18 to get the catalogue, but let's not be fools. We all know who's reading them. The company says it targets the college crowd, but next time you're out, read the logos on the front of sixth-, seventh-, and eighth-graders' clothes. I recently walked into an Abercrombie & Fitch outside of Boston and was greeted at the entrance by a larger-than-life photo of a handsome young man lying on a bed with the zipper to his jeans open at the top. I turned to another store, Express, and watched a shopper about 11 years old pick through thong panties. Some had the word "Sexy" written in rhinestones across the back. No wonder she was looking to buy some—three rear-facing mannequins were displaying them in various colors.

Then, of course, there's television. When's the last time you watched the WB channel and the programs it targets at your kids? Take a look at *Dawson's Creek* or *Buffy the Vampire Slayer*. In fact, try to find an episode in which sex is *not* a central theme. Here are some other suggestions for the concerned and adventurous parent: Watch an MTV video. Or listen to the lyrics on one of the CDs your child plays over and over in his or her portable CD player. Our kids are drowning in sexual messages.

PARENTS: EXHAUSTED AND DISCOURAGED

When our children are young, we're careful to match their toys and experiences to their age. You wouldn't give a 3-year-old a 500-piece puzzle, for instance, or a put a make-your-own-beaded-jewelry set in the hands of a toddler. We turn the TV on to *Sesame Street* or *Mr. Roger's Neighborhood*, not MTV, and pop only a Barney or Disney video into the VCR.

Why, then, when that same child turns 10, would a parent allow him to see movies appropriate for 14- to 17-year-olds? Or let 8-year-olds watch television programs that aren't even appropriate for high school seniors? We know this activity is harmful to them. One study found that more than three out of four Americans felt that the way TV programs show sex encourages irresponsible sexual behavior.[4]

I believe that, as parents, we simply run out of steam. Or we back out of our kids' lives fearing we're being too oppressive, overbearing, or overprotective. Or we mistakenly assume that our kids' minds mature as quickly as their bodies. We assume they can handle messages much like we do. We forget that they perceive and process sexual messages *differently* from the way we do. That's because at different ages, teens are vulnerable to different influences. A 12-year-old and a 15-year-old receive and process the same information in different ways. All teens proceed through cognitive and psychological development at different times. Some mature quickly, others take much longer. We make a terrible mistake if we believe that a 13-year-old will handle sexual messages in the same way a 16-year-old does.

Now, look at what messages we're exposing them to when we give our kids free and open access to all media.

Blockbuster Sex on the Big Screen

Although PG-13 movies are supposed to be restricted from viewing until a child has reached the junior high school level, in reality, 9-, 10-, and 11-year-olds often make up the audience. PG-13 movies target the preadolescent and young teen populations for the same reason advertisers target them—they're easy to hook. This audience is impressionable and easily excitable (particularly when it comes to sexual innuendo). And kids watch movies not once, but repeatedly. Too many parents take this issue lightly. They allow their young children to watch PG-13 or even R-rated movies either because they believe the images of sex and violence won't affect their kids, or because they're simply too tired to argue. The kids, of course, want to be allowed to do anything that their older peers can do, especially if it's something "forbidden."

The reason for talking about "age appropriateness" is that young teens perceive film content in a fundamentally different way from you, I, or even older teens. Consider the impressions they're likely to take away from a film such as *Titanic*. Do kids even remember that the movie was based on a true historical event? Do they remember the old couple who held each other as the ship sank so they could die in each other's arms? The captain who shut himself in his cabin to go down with his ship? Of course not. Kids remember the steamy windows of the car parked below-deck in which Jack and Rose made passionate love. Did she get pregnant? Herpes? Chlamydia? No. She got the "strength" from this three-day tryst to "go on."

The Sounds of Sex: Music and MTV

Turn on the radio and listen to any hip-hop station or any hard rock station. Choose one at random. Then listen to a song...*any* song. I challenge you to find one that doesn't make explicit sexual references. You're also likely to hear lots of vulgar language, racial references, demeaning of women, and glorification of violence, so be prepared.

You need to take this seriously. Music has a huge influence in kids' lives. Research clearly shows that kids who listen to heavy metal music (mostly boys) are more likely to engage in risky behaviors, such as violence, drinking, taking drugs, and having sex. It's no wonder. Kids tune into music so much that it can become their entire world. According to a Kaiser Family Foundation study, young people spend an average of almost an hour and a half a day listening to CDs, tapes, or radio. "After TV, music is the medium of choice for most kids, especially older teens," said Donald F. Roberts, Jr., Ph.D., professor of communication at Stanford University and an author of the Kaiser study, *Kids & Media @ The New Millennium*, which examined media use among a nationally representative sample of more than 3000 children ages 2 to 18.[5]

Remember also that kids no longer simply listen to music; they also watch it on cable channels such as MTV, which is particularly popular with boys. Research shows that 75% of concept videos (those that tell a story) use sexual imagery. In fact, a report by the Center for Media and Public Affairs found that music videos contained more sex per minute than any other media genre.[6] Additionally, one study found that more than half of music videos involve violence—usually against women. Overall, the videos present sex as violent and detached from romance or love.

Don't just wonder what's been playing in your kids' earphones. Listen to their CDs and tapes. Watch MTV with them long enough to get a feel for the variety of videos. Ask your teen why he likes a particular song or band, and listen, really listen, to his answers. But don't be foolish enough to believe him if he says he doesn't listen to the words or only likes the beat.

Many kids will simply shrug their shoulders and answer, "I dunno. I just like it" when you ask for an opinion. The truth is that he may not really know why he likes it, so make him figure it out. Press him with questions that will challenge him to think about what he's watching. This works so much better than simply saying, "That stuff's trash, what in the world are you watching it for?"—an approach that automatically puts him on the defensive, turning him and the artist into allies and you into the enemy.

Personally, I screen music—along with movies and TV shows— pretty carefully and help my own teens figure out what is acceptable and what isn't. As they mature, they have more choices, but I don't let raunchy lyrics into my house. There's plenty of better stuff available.

Don't be afraid to use the same strategy. Boycott objectionable music, movies, or programs in your home, regardless of your teen's age. Many parents don't enforce restrictions because they fear that their kids will rebel. Put your fears away and be honest with your sons and daughters. You don't have to behave like a tyrant and issue commands. Just tell them how you feel about their music and state unequivocally that you won't let it into your home. However much they may argue or sulk, you need to know that your opinions can have a very positive effect on them and their behavior, and in the end, your honesty will make you their role model.

Television: The 800-Pound Gorilla

Our kids are exposed to more television than to any other media. Studies find that most teenagers watch 17 hours of television a week. By the time they graduate high school, they will have spent 12,000 hours in the classroom, but 15,000 hours watching television.[7] Many of them watch alone, in their bedrooms.

No big deal, you think? Well consider that two-thirds (68%) of all programs on television contained sexual content during the 1999/2000 season, a *12%* increase in just two years![8] It's probably much higher now. And here's another interesting statistic: just 1% of people shown having sex are married to each other. That means that 99% of sex that teens see on television occurs between unmarried people. Depictions of sexual acts other than intercourse or fondling have also dramatically increased over the past two decades. On television today, teens are exposed to homosexual sex, oral sex, and multiple partner sex. While overt depictions of these practices are less frequent than those of "traditional sex," references to them are still frequently made.

There are clear connections between what kids see on television and how they behave in real life. An April 2002 survey on teens, sex, and TV from the Kaiser Family Foundation found that nearly three out of four teenagers (72%) thought sex on TV influenced the sexual behavior of kids their age "somewhat" or "a lot." Ironically, just one in four said it influenced their own sexual behavior, while six in ten said television taught them how to say no to a sexual situation that makes them uncomfortable. I have to question that second statistic, however, since the same study found that few young people can cite any role models on television when it comes to sexual decision making.[9]

Many parents believe they can feel secure in allowing their kids unsupervised viewing time during "family hour" at night, that is, the period right after dinner, between 8 and 9 P.M. Unfortunately, such is not the case. That one hour of programming contains an average of eight sexual incidents. In case you harbor any illusions about the general trend in television programming, this figure has *quadrupled* since 1976.[10]

Sex is depicted more explicitly on cable television, but staying with noncable networks won't get you very far. Take the television program *Ally McBeal*, popular in the late 1990s and early 2000s. In one episode, Ally makes an urgent after-hours call to the head of her law firm, Richard Fish. We find him in his bedroom, where he's in bed with Whipper Cone, a judge with whom he has an ongoing relationship. The two are engaged in a flurry of frantic, conjoined movement, bouncing around the bed as the phone continues ringing. Finally, Whipper answers the call. Ally is surprised to recognize Whipper's voice and to hear Richard's moaning in the background. Ally asks for Richard but Whipper says, "He's a little busy right now. Can I have him call you back?" Ally hangs up with a disgusted look on her face while Richard and Whipper continue their sexual episode.[11]

Any teenage boy who happened to be watching this episode has been told something about what sex is like and where it fits into a man's life. Here's what he sees: Richard is successful because he is a lawyer. He's powerful because he is the head of his law firm. He's single and highly sexually charged—even a phone call can't stop his sexual activity. He has no modesty because he doesn't care if the person on the phone hears him.

Now you have been excited and titillated, and you have formed an idea about how successful grown men handle their sex lives. If you're that adolescent boy, with no previous sexual experience, this information is hard to dismiss because it is exciting and interesting. In fact, it has changed you. At school the next day you look at your female classmates differently. You somehow feel more worldly than you did the day before. It's as if you're seeing life through the eyes of Richard Fish. Suddenly the girls around you have all become potential Whippers. You consider asking one of your female classmates out on a date, not so much because you enjoy her company, but because you wonder what it might be like to have sex with her. Or, you could skip the dating altogether and ask if she wants to "hook up"—you saw two young, sophisticated singles in another show do that after they met in a bar.

Here's the problem. You're as young as 14 or maybe as old as 17. If you start having sex now, chances are excellent that you'll become another statistic in the epidemic. You'll get an STD—or two or three. You may put yourself at higher risk for depression as well. And the development of your sexuality? Your masculinity may be fashioned after what you saw in television characters rather than what you've observed among the real (nontelevision) men around you.

I might be accused of exaggerating in the above scenario, but teenage boys and girls are spending more time with television, movies, and music than they are with their parents or other adult role models. Media and the Internet offer our kids around-the-clock sexual training. And they're training them right into a deadly epidemic.

Dotcom Sex

Almost one-third of kids age 10 to 17 with computers at home have seen a pornographic Web site, and not necessarily on purpose. There are many, many ways that you can end up at those sites by accident. A study by the Safe American Foundation reported that 91% of teenagers said they unintentionally accessed Web sites featuring pornographic, hate-based, or violent material while conducting research for school or just surfing the Web.[12]

Now, knowing this, and knowing that Internet pornography can be harmful, or even traumatic, for your teen, not to mention the fact that pedophiles and sexually addicted adults frequently log on posing as teens, you need to know where your child has been online and what he or she has been doing there. How do you find out? Ask. Then get on your computer and follow his or her tracks. If you don't know how, ask an Internet-savvy friend.

Don't be surprised if you find yourself wondering why in the world your teen talked you into having a laptop or PC in his room. Now is the time to talk yourself back out of it. Keep your computer and Internet access in a public spot in your home so that your teen won't get into trouble. It's a very simple move and can save a lot of heartache for families.

Selling Shampoo... or Sex?

Advertising companies use sexual imagery to sell our kids on everything from shampoo to clothing to athletic shoes. Sexually seductive messages are pervasive in television and magazine ads, in which young girls are made up and dressed to appear several years older than they actually are. They do this because it works. We all remember the Calvin Klein ads on TV. Many adults objected to them, but they sold jeans by the ton.

One researcher of media influences has made an astute observation. He noted that while advertisers use sex to sell numerous products to our kids, and those kids respond to sexual cues and begin sexual activity at an early age, our society blames the kids rather than the advertisers.[13] This may not exactly be blaming the victim for the crime, but it comes very close. After all, it's the advertisers who assault the senses of the kids, not the other way around.

A teenage girl can pass by almost any clothing store in any mall and see huge posters of midget-sized bikinis on laughing teen girls embraced by well-built young men with low-slung pants. The teen thinks it's a cool poster, so she buys a tiny bikini. She goes to the beach and gets a lot of stares from teen boys, but also a lot of comments from adults who say that she's acting immodestly. All she did, in reality, was respond exactly the way advertisers wanted her to—she bought their product. And given the fact that she's a little impulsive and very impressionable, as most teenagers naturally are, we might even say she's been manipulated.

TEENS: SOAKING IT UP LIKE A SPONGE

No discussion of teen sex would be complete without a detailed understanding of the impact of sexual messages (whether through words or visual imagery) on the tender adolescent psyche. And the impact is profound. The adolescent brain is like a huge bed of raw nerve endings waiting to soak up messages that come its way.

Overall, a teen instinctively relates incoming messages to his or her self-image much more readily than an adult would, primarily because the teen mind is extremely egocentric. The psychological theory related to this, called Berkowitz's cognitive neoassociationist theory, says that when you have an emotional response to certain information, you behave according to that emotional response. Thus, if a sexual scene on TV leaves a teenager feeling romantic, and he or she likes that feeling, he or she may act out that behavior because of the pleasant emotional response.

Those emotional responses may not lead to sexual acts until months or perhaps years after the message is received, but eventually it occurs. This is particularly true for many of our teens who are emotionally adrift, lonely, and in desperate search of a meaningful identity. They are particularly vulnerable to sexual images because, unlike adults, they lack both the real-life experience and complete cognitive development to make judgments based on anything *but* an immediate emotional response.

You and I filter messages we receive through a gauntlet of memories and lessons learned, which helps determine whether they're acted upon or rejected. Teenagers have no such filter. Most 10- to 13-year-olds don't have a long history of sexual experiences. So when they're exposed to sexual images, sexual talk, or sexual lyrics, the messages are fresh and exciting. Young adolescents have no frame of reference with which to assess these messages. They may feel sexually aroused by what they hear and see, but they don't know what to do with this feeling or how to understand it.

When a young girl, for example, watches a movie scene in which a man behaves both violently and sexually toward a woman, she has no idea if this reflects the reality of everyday life. So let's say a 14-year-old girl watches an older guy shoving and pushing a woman on the screen, only to force her arms behind her back, slam her hard against a wall, and then start to force himself on her sexually. The woman on the screen—because she's only acting—responds to him with obvious enjoyment.

Now our young girl thinks that what's going on in the movie is acceptable. The woman on the screen didn't cry, so it couldn't have really hurt, and as the camera fades, it's obvious that the two went on to have intercourse. So what does our 14-year-old think as she leaves the theater? That mixing violence and sex is okay. What should she expect when she goes out on her first date? She doesn't know, but a few more episodes like the one she just saw will lead her to believe that if a guy does that to *her*, it's "okay" too. You'd be surprised at how often girls put up with physical abuse from their boyfriends and never tell their parents.

The Three Lessons

There are three primary lessons teenagers learn from the hundreds of thousands of sexual messages they're exposed to:
1. Sex is BIG
2. Sexuality is the largest dimension of a person's personality
3. Cool people are promiscuous
Let's explore each.

SEX IS BIG

When a national disaster like September 11 occurs, the intense media focus on the event gives us the sense that, at the moment, this is one of the most important things in our lives. The same thing happens with sex in the media. The constant attention the media focuses on sex means it occupies a place of disproportionate importance in the lives of our kids. Given the sheer numbers of sexual messages that assault our kids daily, it's no surprise that sex seems to them to loom like Mt. Everest in the center of their lives.

This is a dangerous state of mind because it comes at a time when adolescents are trying to sort through and understand their place in the world, a time in which they're trying to bring a semblance of order to lives that often feel chaotic and disordered. Some serious issues arise when sexual activity is drummed into teenagers as *disproportionately important.*

First, they have to figure out if and how to integrate this imposing sexual force into their lives. Their solutions, of course, are profoundly influenced by their overall emotional development and sexuality. If a teen feels emotionally strong and stable, he can decipher sexual messages more clearly and integrate them into his life in a way that is healthy and comfortable. A teen who is developing a strong sense of identity, feels good about who he is, and, most importantly, feels affirmed by his parents is unlikely to be enticed into sexual activity by media images. But if he doesn't know who he is, if he feels unloved and empty inside, his neediness and his emotional vulnerability make him much more receptive to toxic sexual messages. Likewise, if he's emotionally insecure or has negative feelings about his sexuality, he may integrate sexual messages into his life in a very unhealthy way.

Anna, a 16-year-old patient of mine, is an inspiring example of someone who stays out of sexual trouble because of her strong sense of identity. Anna lives with her divorced mother and younger sister. She's always been very close to her mother, and the two spend a lot of time together, talking about everything. Anna says her mother is "strict."

Still, when we discussed what she watched on television, what magazines she read, or what music she listened to, all her choices contained a lot of sexual material. So I asked her if she thought about becoming sexually active. "No way," she said in a determined voice. "Not until I'm much older." When I asked how she came to that decision, she said her mom told her she was way too valuable. She was smart and had a future. Her body, which would carry her into that future, was important and should be respected.

I could tell by her tone that she believed her mother. I wondered out loud what she thought of all the sex in movies, magazines, and songs. The women in the soap operas and on the magazine covers, she said, were "all messed up." Even as she watched women jump from man to man and one bed to another, she knew this was not a healthy lifestyle. But she continued to watch because the shows "hooked her." She needed to find out from day to day who was going to cheat on whom. She could even recite how frequently she saw sex on her soaps.

While these highly sexual shows may have hooked Anna's curiosity, she was able to remove herself from their implicit messages, drawing strength from something bigger and more important in her life—her relationship with her mother and, very significantly, her mother's appreciation of her. She talked with her mom about life, school, friends, and boys. She and her mother respected each other. They weren't best buddies, but she knew she could rely on her mom for anything. This healthy self-esteem, connection with her mother, and strong sense of who she was enabled Anna to integrate these messages in her life, but keep them, very appropriately, quite small.

Sex Symbols as Role Models

Blowing sex out of proportion also encourages kids to identify with "sex symbols" in the media. Here's how it happens.

Many teens go through a stage of development during which they imagine people are constantly watching them and may even know what they're thinking. Of course this is not true, but it feels true to them. In essence, teens feel that they have relationships with people that they may in fact really not have.

This may sound crazy to adults, but this state of mind is quite common in teens. Imagine how this developmental phase could "help" a teen who is very lonely. To comfort himself, all he needs to do is develop a couple of imaginary friendships. Television provides ample opportunity for him to choose his "friendships" because the men and women he sees on the screen are more glamorous and sexy than people in real life. He can fantasize what it would be like to hang out with them, and may even have conjured up "conversations" with them.

The real danger is that, after attachments are formed, vulnerable teens may be likely to imitate the behavior of their new-found friends, which often means becoming sexually active or even promiscuous.

Tony, 15, is a good example. He struggles in school because of his attention-deficit disorder, but he's popular and outgoing. His parents, like Anna's, are divorced. When I asked what he watched on television and what kind of music he listened to, he described movies and music with highly charged sexual content. I asked what he thought about them, and he looked at me like I was an idiot. Of course he watched and listened because of the sex, he said. The more he watched, the more he wanted to watch.

"Do you have a girlfriend?" I asked.

"Of course," he replied. Not a romantic girlfriend, he said, but he'd had sex with several girls. When I asked about important relationships in his life, he said he considered his friends more important to him than his mother or siblings. His peers understood him better. As I probed, I found he spent extremely little time each week with his mother. He had no grandparents, aunts, or uncles with whom he could connect. As we spoke about his life and relationships, I could hear his voice harden and his tone become distant. Clearly, the lack of substantive adult relationships caused him pain, so he turned where he could—to friends, movies, and music—to fill the empty spaces.

In doing so, he integrated sexual messages into his life in very unhealthy ways. Because he was so emotionally vulnerable, he sopped these messages up like a sponge. He also formed intense attachments to musicians on music videos, fantasizing that he was intimately connected with them. Tony, like so many teen boys, looked around to male role models to try to figure out what maleness was all about. What he found was men singing raunchy music lyrics.

He needed male friends—and there they were, singing to Tony through the TV screen. And Tony responded. They became his imaginary friends. He began to talk like them. He wore clothes like theirs. He even wanted to take up the electric guitar at an older age, fantasizing that he might one day join the band. Forming such attachments is a well-known psychological mechanism adolescents use to cope with loneliness, emptiness, confusion, and depression.

A Force Beyond Their Control

Finally, if sex is such an imposing force, teens may feel they don't have the means to control it. This is particularly true with our teen boys. We, as a collective adult culture, treat our adolescent boys as if they're helpless in the face of their own sexual drives. We communicate clearly—through our language and even in sex education classes—that we don't expect boys to control themselves. Handing teen boys condoms says, "I know you can't say no to sex, so use this."

We saw earlier that healthy identity formation and character development depend on teens learning to become responsible and independent. Central to this development is the issue of control. Teens must learn to internalize rules, boundaries, and authority in order to control their decisions and behaviors. As children, they depend on external factors like parents and teachers to set and enforce the rules and help them control their behavior. The healthy transition to adulthood depends upon their being able to assert control themselves. But when they perceive that there is a huge part of their character that shouldn't or can't be controlled, their psychological maturity is brought to a screeching halt. Many adolescent psychiatrists have long advocated the importance of learning control over one's sexual impulses as crucial to sound character development. As *The Harvard Guide to Modern Psychiatry* notes: "Sexual impulses intensify during puberty, remain intense during this phase of adolescence. Permissiveness, the lack of moral guidelines, the sexually stimulating aspects of the mass media, and other dimensions of today's society make control of these impulses particularly difficult for the modern adolescent. . . . How the adolescent handles these conflicting internal and external demands determines in large measure his future character structure. His ability to attain impulse control will determine the extent of this control as an adult." Furthermore, the authors conclude, " . . . sexual freedom has a destructive effect on an adolescent's ability to sublimate sexual impulses and establish a mature character structure." [14] And, in fact, this inability to control these sexual desires sends many adolescents seeking help from psychiatrists and other therapists.

Teens who fear that they cannot control their sexual impulses may fear that they cannot control other impulses as well. In fact, they wonder what in the world they can control. Learning impulse control is an integral part of adult psychological development, and sabotaging it by teaching kids they can't control their sexual behavior does them a terrible disservice and leaves them feeling as if they have no solid emotional ground to stand on.

I've seen this among my own patients. Girls who have numerous sexual partners have described to me an underlying chaos in their lives. Many drink, stay out all hours of the night, and do poorly in school. They have difficulty pointing to any part of their life where they feel in charge. Everything seems to be falling in around them. I am convinced that these young girls are terrified. They are frightened by chaos and they are frightened because they feel that they have no emotional or psychological resources to pull any part of their lives into order. They feel out of control and their lives reflect it.

SEXUALITY IS THE LARGEST DIMENSION OF A PERSON'S PERSONALITY

If your wife or husband commented on your weight each day, you would begin to believe that your weight was important to him or her, maybe more important than other aspects of your life and personality. The same thing happens with sex. When the media applauds sex more than substantive character qualities or natural talent, teens deduce that sex is, therefore, a more important part of their identity than their own intellect, natural abilities, or character. For instance, young girls see pictures of busty, sexy women. They see women talking about how to have sex with men, about sexual techniques and orgasms. They don't see articles about girls' IQ, athletic abilities, or patience. Professional women scientists, politicians, and poets don't grace the covers of magazines or provide the voice-overs for perfume ads on television. Some star female athletes have appeared in TV advertisements for credit cards, makeup, and even financial advising companies, but it's clear from the ad that they're capitalizing on their sexuality rather than their sports prowess to sell the product.

Teens will instinctively try music or sports, and experiment with different groups of friends in an effort to figure out what they're good at and what they're not. When a teen looks around, he doesn't see a constant stream of messages about the intrinsic value of his musical talent, his intellectual curiosity, sports abilities, or good friendships. The big payoff for everything is sex. The top athletes, business people, politicians, and artists get to have sex whenever and with whomever they wish. All their talents and achievements have no value in themselves. They seem to be in the service of sex. That's the message.

In this context, how can teens not feel that their sexuality and sexual interest are more important than their talents, gifts, and character?

Even if a young girl has a wonderful artistic talent, she begins to doubt herself if it doesn't make her "sexier," that is, lead to a more active sex life.

Teen boys are also vulnerable to this message. Many strive to bolster their sense of identity through athletics. A boy who enjoys biking may follow Lance Armstrong's performance intensely. He looks to Lance as an admirable, strong man and finds that he, too, can bike pretty well. So he works at it. He enters races and finds that he comes close to winning some. His confidence in himself builds and he likes what's happening. But when he flips on the television, Lance isn't the guy he sees. Instead, he sees models, actors, and rock stars in highly sexed situations with beautiful women. More attention is given to sexual prowess than to athletic pursuits. He may easily come to feel that what he has to offer the world is worthless. He may even decide to give up biking and devote his time to the pursuit of sex. Or he may suffer a depression.

We shouldn't tolerate this situation. We need to begin giving media time to, and talking about, the dimensions of our teen boys that are really important—their character, their giftedness, their athletic talents, and their intellectual gifts. Why? Because *these* are the reasons that we love our sons and brothers and spouses. Young men need to know that they are loved for who they are, not because they are sexual.

COOL PEOPLE ARE PROMISCUOUS

Any good teacher knows that modeling behavior is the best way to teach teenagers how to act. Teens watch, listen, and wait, then watch again. They're keenly attuned to our moods and feelings because their feelings (and sometimes behaviors) depend on cues they receive from us and from other adults in their lives. And kids love to imitate the behavior they see. They size up what they see, mimic it, and if they like it, incorporate it into their lives. These observations have been formalized into something called Bandura's observational learning theory, which teaches that children respond particularly well to role models they admire and with whom they identify.

We see Bandura's theory at work in the response of teen girls to media images, such as Jennifer Aniston's haircut on *Friends*. Girls admired Jennifer's behavior, personality, and appearance and wanted to identify more closely with her. So many got their hair cut to look just like hers. Our generation did the same thing 20 years ago when we mimicked ice skater Dorothy Hamill's wedge cut.

To take the theory to its logical conclusion, if kids cut their hair like celebrities, they won't for a moment hesitate to imitate their flirtatious and sexual behavior as well.

Bandura's theory suggests that "children will learn not only the mechanics of sexual behavior, but the contexts, motives and consequences portrayed. They will attend to and learn from models who are attractive, powerful, rewarded, and similar to themselves." A Kaiser Family Foundation report found this was true, noting that while "children do not usually act immediately on what they learn from television . . . they store such knowledge to be used when their own circumstances elicit it."[15]

Now, think about the popular shows that teens watch. Think about the many sophisticated, beautiful, sexual men and women who draw our kids to the TV set in hordes. Bandura's theory teaches us that somewhere in the psyches of our kids are stored images, feelings, and beliefs about these men and women and what they're doing sexually. Teens decide whether they like what they see or not, and keep it in a psychological reservoir to be retrieved whenever they feel a need to use it. A 13-year-old, for instance, might admire Madonna's seductively aggressive behavior but be afraid to imitate her just yet. If she likes what she sees, however, she will tuck her feelings and images of the singer away and retrieve them when she is ready to imitate them—which may be one, two, even three years later.

Thus, teens are constantly absorbing new ways of thinking and acting. This, coupled with their strong desire to "fit in" to their peer group, can be a dangerous formula when it comes to sexual messages.

SO WHAT ARE PARENTS TO DO?

Selling sex to teens is just as bad as selling them cigarettes and alcohol. Can you imagine the public outrage of parents if movies, magazines, and music incorporated glamorous smoking imagery to the same degree they do sexual content? Or if advertisers used cigarettes to sell their jeans, shampoos, and soaps? Imagine this occurring in the midst of an epidemic of lung diseases among teens! Parents, teachers, and physicians would pressure Congress day and night.

Well, this is *exactly* what is occurring with the sexual content in our media and our teens. Only instead of an epidemic of lung diseases, we have an epidemic of sexually transmitted diseases.

Many researchers suggest that adults must lobby strongly for more realistic sexual messages, that we must force Congress to pass legislation requiring films and TV shows to include references to sexual risks and ways to avoid them in programs that have sexual content. I would like to see Congress go a step farther. I would like to see legislation that bans all sexual content from advertising, movies, and magazines promoted to teenage and younger audiences. Prime-time television should not include sexual content. Movies rated PG-13 should not have sexually explicit content, whether or not they make reference to contraception.

Until we become angry enough to fight the entertainment industry and pressure our federal government to protect our children from having sex sold to them, the madness will continue.

KEEP YOUR STANDARDS HIGHER THAN HOLLYWOOD'S

You don't have to wait for Congress. There are actions that you, as a parent or concerned adult, can take today. If Hollywood rates a movie PG-13, follow the rating to the letter. A PG-13 rating means a child should be 13 before viewing the movie. If the movie is rated R (requiring a parent or guardian if the child is under 17), make your 16-year-old wait. And don't, as an alternative, offer to sit and watch restricted movies with your child. Regardless of what is said afterward, the simple act of watching it will sanction the movie and its content in your teen's mind.

When teens understand that a parent's motives are genuine and rooted in love, they'll accept an enormous amount. If a young teen— and even an older one—sees his parents expend time and energy to teach him about his mind and emotions, that teen feels wonderful and valuable. He may complain that his parents are overprotective, but deep down, he feels cherished.

Discussing with your teenager the sexual content of movies and the harm it can cause helps them realize you're on their side. So ask your teenager what *he* thinks is appropriate in movies and why. Then ask what he thinks is bad and why. Ask how he felt when he saw sex in a television show and then ask if he felt it was realistic. By questioning teens, we can help them come to conclusions on their own about what is acceptable and what is not.

I find that when teens (particularly girls) understand the motives of the media moguls in incorporating so much sexuality into their products—namely, to sell their wares to teens—they become angry. They feel used and exploited. Igniting teens to rebel against that which they feel is using them and causing them harm is highly effective. It's working with cigarette smoking and it can work with sexuality in the media. Teach them to be smart, to refuse to accept garbage into their brilliant minds. Teach them that they are far too valuable for that "stuff."

Finally, fight fire with fire. The motive behind the explosion of sexual content in media and advertising is money, so money can be our weapon. While mass media and big business are much richer than most of us, we still control the buying power. Boycott those who are the worst offenders. We are parents—we are reality. What we have to offer is truth, love, and wisdom. As much as the media tries hard to take life away from our kids, we have the authority and means to give it back. *We have the power!*

NINE

■ In a national survey, 26% of sexually active 15- to 17-year-olds surveyed said one "cannot become infected with HIV by having unprotected oral sex."

High-Risk Sex

IN 1996, THE SMALL, UPSCALE community of Conyers, Georgia, experienced an epidemic of syphilis. More than 200 teenagers—many as young as 13 and 14—were infected. When officials and the media investigated, they discovered a community in which teens gathered in large, empty houses for drinking, drugs, and group sex. A small core of teens had had sex with as many as 50 different people in a short span of time (one young girl told health officials she'd slept with at least 65 people). Some of them had been holding "study groups," in which they watched, then re-enacted scenes from The Playboy Channel in their bedrooms. Preteen girls admitted to participating in an act they called "the sandwich," in which one girl had oral sex with a boy while having vaginal sex with another boy and anal sex with a third boy, all at the same time. The girls also had sex with each other.[1,2]

When we hear stories like this, we become appropriately horrified, but we also smugly assume that our teens are too smart to get involved in this kind of behavior. Hopefully, yours are that smart, but one thing is certain: Even if they aren't involved, they have at some time felt the pressure to participate and they hear about sex between other kids frequently. Maybe they've even seen others in a sex act. I know this because I hear it from so many patients in my own practice. We, as parents, have a responsibility to understand these pressures so that we can help our kids get through them.

The world of sex your kids know isn't the one you knew. It's broader, colder, and far more shocking than anything we ever dreamed of in the 1960s. Anal sex. Group sex. Voyeuristic sex. Heterosexual vaginal intercourse, homosexual sex, and bisexual sex. Oral sex in public places—including schools! I listen to the stories every day in my office. And just when I think I've heard about the most peculiar sexual encounter I could possibly imagine, I hear an even more bizarre and disturbing one. Consider:

• Of 1067 teens aged 13 to 18 surveyed in the early 1980s, roughly one-fifth (20%) said they had ever had oral sex. But ten years later, that figure had jumped to 70% of males and 57% of females who'd had oral sex even *before* they had actual intercourse.[3]

• In 1992, a study of a group of ninth- through twelfth-graders revealed that nearly a third of those who were still virgins had engaged in masturbation with a partner.[4]

• In a 2000 survey by the Kaiser Family Foundation, one in five teens reported that oral sex is "safe sex."[5]

• A 2000 Special Report in *Family Planning Perspectives* revealed that in a volunteer sample of 311 nonvirgin college undergraduates, 70% of boys and 57% percent of girls reported having performed oral sex at least once before their first intercourse. And 57 to 58% of both boys and girls reported receiving oral sex before intercourse. The same report also revealed that in a 1992 HIV prevention program in Los Angeles, 29 to 31% of 2026 ninth- through twelfth-grade virgins reported having engaged in masturbation with a partner. What's more, many of these teens said they do not consider mutual masturbation or oral sex to be sex—some even call oral sex and mutual masturbation "abstinence"![6]

It's no doubt, the new "styles" and ways of sex among teens are fueling the epidemic.

WHY IT'S HAPPENING

There are many reasons for this eruption in high-risk sexual behaviors. Just think back to the late 1990s, when President Clinton publicly declared "I did not have sex with that woman." The Monica Lewinski scandal gave new meaning to the word "sex," and taught an entire nation of teenagers that as long as you didn't have "vaginal penetration," you really weren't having "sex."

Also, because we are such a sexually explicit and open country, many kids are encouraged to push the envelope as far as they can when it comes to sexual experimentation. I've seen the results among my patients. The more kids experiment, the more quickly they become bored with sex, and the more they search for another thrill, a newer excitement, like drug addicts who need more and more poison to get the high they crave. Lest you think this is happening only in urban areas or among disadvantaged people, I recently interviewed a teacher in a large Midwestern city located in the heart of the Bible belt. I asked if she'd seen any changes in sexual activity and sexual talk among her high school students during the 20 years she'd been teaching. Her moan of despair caught me by surprise.

"Oral sex," she said.

"What do you mean?" I asked.

She described a note she'd recently found on her classroom floor from a ninth-grade boy in her class. It read: "Sorry I didn't get to the bathroom at noon for my blow job. I forgot today was taco day in the cafeteria." No intimacy expressed. Just the basic sense that sex wasn't worth giving up tacos for. I hope this disturbs you as much as it does me and this young man's teacher. But the teacher wasn't finished yet. "Kids have oral sex in *groups!*" She almost screamed the words at me. "Sometimes kids meet after a movie. The boys line up and different girls go down the line giving them oral sex. Together—in front of each other. I just don't get it. They're great kids. But they're going wild over oral sex. They think they're safe and they really believe they're not having sex—hard to believe, isn't it?"

Yes, it is hard to believe that our own children would be doing this sort of thing, but they are. In great numbers.

ORAL SEX: A CRAZE WITH CONSEQUENCES

News about a new fad of oral sex among teenagers and even oral sex parties first filtered into my office about three years ago. I knew it was on the rise around the country when Elayne Bennett (wife of William Bennett, former secretary of education in the Reagan administration, and later national drug czar) phoned me to ask about transmission of STDs through oral sex in order to prepare for a television dialogue with ex-Surgeon General Joycelyn Elders. This occurred during the summer of 1999. I told Elayne that the risk of contracting STDs by having sex this way is extremely high. Interestingly, as I watched Joycelyn Elders talk about teen sexual behavior during the program, she seemed to be backing away from her advocacy of condom distribution to teens and agreed that teaching teens abstinence from sex was a good thing. In short, even she seemed surprised about the increased intensity of teen sexual behavior and the "alternate" behaviors they were adopting in order to avoid pregnancy.

Over the next couple of years, I began questioning teens about what was going on among their friends and in their schools. One phrase kept coming up over and over: oral sex. I began calling teachers and school counselors in my area, then around the country to put my finger on the pulse of changing sexual behaviors among kids. Was what had happened in Georgia simply an isolated event? Or was it the symptom of a larger problem, as I suspected? I felt angry. I felt scared. But I also felt motivated. I decided that parents and others need to know what I found out about what our kids are up to, and why.

In my own practice, I'm so accustomed to seeing junior high school students who have engaged in fellatio or cunnilingus that I no longer simply ask if they're sexually active. I always ask specifically about oral sex, as well.

I ask because I've learned that kids think they're safe if they adopt an "anything but intercourse" approach to sex. For instance, the *Family Planning Perpectives* report cites one study of 600 Midwestern college students, which found that nearly six out of ten (59%) did not believe oral sex qualified as sex, and 19% thought anal sex was not really sex.[7] Interestingly, girls were more likely than boys to say that oral sex was not sex. Also, these same students were less likely to identify couples as "sexual partners" if they exclusively participated in oral sex rather than intercourse. With oral sex, kids think they can avoid pregnancy and diseases while still enjoying the pleasures of sexual activity and retaining their virginity, which is extremely important to them. An online survey conducted by *Twist* magazine found that of the 10,000 girls who responded, eight out of ten said they were virgins, even though one-fourth of the "virgins" had had oral sex. Over half of the respondents (5,700) were under 14 years old![8]

ORAL SEX IS NO PROTECTION

You can mince words all you like, but while oral sex may leave you a technical virgin, it won't leave you disease-free. Unfortunately, too few kids understand this.

In a national survey of teens conducted for the Kaiser Family Foundation, 26% of sexually active 15- to 17-year-olds surveyed said one "cannot become infected with HIV by having unprotected oral sex," and an additional 15% didn't know whether or not they could become infected. The sad truth is that HIV *is* spread through oral sex, as are herpes, syphilis, gonorrhea, HPV, chancroid, intestinal parasites, and hepatitis A.[9, 10]

Beyond the physical ramifications of oral sex are the emotional ones, especially for psychologically immature or confused teenagers. Oral sex is intimate and private, and involves exposing a very personal, special part of the self to another person. It's not like kissing or petting with your clothes on. It can put a young person into a position of extreme emotional vulnerability and can leave him or her feeling used and abused.

I particularly worry about girls who engage in fellatio (and experts believe there's a lot more fellatio going on than cunnilingus).[11] What will go through their minds in 20 years when they're married and have children? Will their memories become painful, even traumatic reminders for them? Or will they forget their encounters, and push them into the recesses of their hearts as they struggle not to remember? One thing is certain: For most of these girls, these will not be memories they will cherish into adulthood.

Mary Ellen's Story

I'd known Mary Ellen for nine years when she came in for her annual physical at age 15. She had always been a highly impressionable girl, given to extreme mood swings. She was easily manipulated because she was a people-pleaser, and she especially craved the attention of men and boys. She had always had a volatile relationship with her father, partly because he didn't know how to deal with her impulsive behavior and moodiness. Sometimes he became so frustrated he locked her in her room, screaming at her that she was a bad kid.

She didn't let any of this get her down, though. Somewhere in Mary Ellen was a fire that wouldn't die. She was impish and playful. She seemed to understand even when she was very young that she was different from other kids in many ways, and miraculously, she accepted and even liked her own unconventionality.

During her physical, I asked all the routine questions. Home life was okay—same old, same old. She couldn't wait to get away and go to college. Boyfriend? Of course, she said, giggling impishly. This one's name was Tyler. A 20-year-old who worked at a garage in town repairing cars, who she thought wonderful.

When I asked if the two of them were sexually active she winced. "No way," she said firmly. I was glad to hear it, but something in her tone bothered me. "You have talked about it with each other, haven't you?" I pressed.

"Oh yeah—and he says he's okay waiting until I'm older or we're married."

Still, something was wrong. I decided to be more specific. "Do you kiss?"

"Of course," she said, blushing.

"Do you go farther than kissing?" I asked, watching her face to see if she was telling me the truth.

"Well, yeah. Sure."

"Do you ever take your clothes off together?" I pressed.

"Well, yeah, it's kind of embarrassing to do and it's embarrassing to talk about." She became more uncomfortable. "What's your favorite thing to do together sexually?" I said.

Without hesitation she responded, "He loves my blow jobs."

"What about you?" I asked. "What do you like?" She seemed surprised by my inquiry.

"Me? Oh, I don't know. I sure don't *like* blow jobs . . . you know what I mean? I guess you'd call it oral sex. I think it's gross."

Here I had two problems on my hands. First, I needed to

re-educate Mary Ellen about what sex was and wasn't. Then I needed to help her untangle her misguided behavior. In desperately wanting affection from Tyler, she allowed him to manipulate her and convince her to engage in behavior she disliked, behavior that was dangerous.

I told her she was at serious risk of getting chlamydia, gonorrhea, herpes, or some other STD. Then I confronted her with some down-and-dirty questions. Did she know whether Tyler was disease-free? She said she hadn't asked. Had she looked at his penis, even casually, to see if he had any sores? She winced as if she were disgusted. You may find my approach too blunt and insensitive, but if you were her doctor and you wanted to know if she had any diseases (or if her boyfriend had), what would you do? My belief is that kids need to know the reality of what they're up against, both for the sake of their own health and to prevent further spread of disease.

What upset me most about Mary Ellen, even more than the threat of disease, was her acting like a sex slave to her boyfriend. She was fulfilling his sexual desires even though she disliked what she was doing, probably even more than she was letting on to me. He was using her with no thought whatsoever for her feelings or her health, and she was going along with it.

I felt like shaking her. But I didn't. I calmly asked why she continued to give Tyler oral sex, even though she didn't like doing it. Aside from the fact that she said it made Tyler happy, she admitted that she didn't really know. She did say one thing, however, that spoke volumes. It was this: "In my school, all the guys expect it and all the girls do it."

Mary Ellen and I spent a lot of time together after that visit. Because of time limitations for office appointments, I rescheduled her again and again. I became determined to help her change her sexual behavior over the next six months if she was agreeable. She was and we did. She began to realize that she didn't have to do anything (particularly something so dangerous) if she didn't want to.

Sadly, the whole concept of taking control of her own behavior was new to her. Her reaction was typical of many girls. They don't feel they really have a choice about sex, particularly about oral sex. Risk of pregnancy used to be an "out" for girls—it was the excuse they used when they didn't want to "go all the way." That risk, condom or not, was one they didn't want. But with oral sex, that risk doesn't exist, and many girls have said that they simply don't know what excuse to give when they feel pressured. They're afraid that if they bring up the subject of disease, their boyfriends will feel insulted.

Once Mary Ellen came to realize that she was in charge of her sexual decisions, she stopped giving Tyler oral sex. And guess what happened to their relationship? Sure enough, he broke it off. At first she felt terribly sad, but after some time went by, she began to realize that he had been dominating and grossly disrespecting her. To be fair, these dynamics were not necessarily intentional on his part. They probably flowed naturally from what she was doing and what he was getting. Oral sex set them up to have an unhealthy relationship.

HOMOSEXUAL SEXUAL ACTIVITY

When teenagers first begin experiencing sexual desires, along with trying to figure out who they are and where they fit into their family structures and peer groups, they may begin experimenting with homosexuality.

Some have a strong predisposition to homosexuality, and are deeply drawn to the same sex in the same way that heterosexual teens are drawn to the opposite sex. Others do it for fun and out of curiosity, or because of a deep emotional conflict with the opposite sex.

Girls who have experienced terror and pain at the hands of a father, uncle, stepfather, or other male adult figure may hate men intensely. Their bad experiences may lead them to repel male affection and drive them toward female affection. Often this happens without their overt awareness.

A teenage boy who desires sex with other boys or men may also have psychological issues with women or even men. He may have felt severely dominated by or disappointed in a woman—perhaps his mother, grandmother, or a sister—who was supposed to love him, but who instead heaped pain and shame on him, making him feel sexually safe only with other men. Or he may have been sexually abused, possibly by a man, resulting in a deep psychic conflict that makes many turn to men and act out sexualized love.

Although there are no solid studies on the numbers of teenage homosexuals nationally, statewide surveys report that between 2 and 5% of teenagers report having experienced some form of homosexual activity.[12] Teen homosexuality is hard to determine for a couple of reasons.

First of all, homosexual experimentation is very common among both boys and girls during early adolescence, and participating in this kind of play does not mean that a kid is homosexual. Perhaps some boys feel more comfortable exploring one another's bodies than they do touching a girl's. Usually these episodes of sexual experimentation are brief and psychologically harmless. The point is, many early pubertal teens experiment with homosexual touch and mature into healthy heterosexuals.

Second, many teens won't divulge information about homosexual interactions because they're embarrassed. They keep their behaviors secret and ponder them. Sexual orientation can be quite confusing for teens because they're going through identity formation. So, if they have an experimental homosexual encounter and are too embarrassed to talk about it, they often wonder if they really are heterosexual or if they have strong homosexual urges. These concerns and questions can remain locked inside their minds and worry the heck out of them.

Regardless of the reason for its happening, homosexual activity, particularly between boys, is extremely dangerous, especially if they engage in anal intercourse. The anus opens into the rectum—the lower end of the large intestine—which is not as well suited for penile penetration as the female vagina is. Both the anus and rectum have rich blood supplies, and their walls, thinner than the walls of the vagina, are easily damaged. When penetration occurs, it's easier to tear blood vessels, which in turn increases the risk of acquiring or receiving an infection as penile skin and/or semen comes in contact with the partner's blood or semen.

There are other risks as well. The anus and rectum can contain potentially dangerous bacteria. For instance, hepatitis A is transmitted through contact with infected feces. Thus, anal intercourse puts sexual partners at higher risk for contracting this disease, which can cause severe liver damage or even kill you. *Shigella* is bacteria found in feces that can also be transmitted through anal intercourse. *Entamoeba* and *Giardia* are two protozoa (single-celled organisms) found in stool, both of which can cause chronic diarrhea. And, of course, there is HIV and hepatitis B. From July 1998 to June 1999, half of all HIV diagnoses among boys age 13 to 19 were attributed to homosexual activity.[13]

Another important factor in the high incidence of STDs in gays is that many have multiple partners. The 1995 Massachusetts Youth Risk Behavior Surveillance found that gay, lesbian, and bisexual orientation was associated with having had sexual intercourse before age 13, with having four or more partners in a lifetime, and with having experienced sexual contact against one's will.[14] Remember: the more partners, the more diseases.

Today, teens are also "coming out" at earlier ages. A few years ago, gay boys and girls tended to announce their sexuality between the

(continued on page 160)

How High the Risk?

The longer a teen can wait to begin sexual activity, the less likely it is that he or she will contract a sexually transmitted disease. Studies show decisively that the earlier a teen begins having sex, the more partners he or she will have. And

Number of sex partners

1

2

3

4

5

6

7

8

9

10

11

12

the more partners, the more exposure to infection. The illustration below shows the number of people teens are exposed to if they have sex with a certain number of partners, and those partners have the same number of partners.

	Number of people exposed to
	1
	3
	7
	15
	31
	63
	127
	255
	511
	1,023
	2,047
	4,095

Adapted from "How at Risk Are You?" from Why kNOw Abstinence Education Programs, Chattanooga, Tenn.

ages of 18 and 22. Today, kids as young as 12 are declaring they're gay.[15] I have two serious concerns about this trend. First, kids at 12 or 13 are still in the process of identity formation. How can they possibly know yet what their sexual orientation will be? Second, and more importantly, younger adolescents, no matter what their sexual orientation, are at high risk for having multiple partners and more diseases if they start having sex at an early age. Gay or straight, these kids are running a great risk.

As we saw in Chapter 5, homosexual teens are also at high risk for depression and suicide. One study published in the *Archives of Pediatric and Adolescent Medicine* found gay or bisexual teenagers are more than three times as likely to attempt suicide as their heterosexual peers.[16]

MORE IS NOT BETTER: MULTIPLE PARTNERS

In both homosexual relationships and heterosexual relationships, teens have been exhibiting a disturbing trend toward sex with multiple partners. Sometimes it happens serially, that is, a teenager has sex with one partner, then another, then another, like an adult going through a series of divorces. But sometimes they have sex with several—or many—partners at once, either concurrently or, like the Conyers teenagers, during group sex.

From what I have learned during interviews with teachers and high school counselors around the country, group sex is more popular with younger teens (particularly at the eighth-grade level). This actually makes sense. Thirteen-year-old kids can't drive, so it's harder for two kids to sneak off to a private place. Also, they lack emotional maturity and may be more easily titillated by sex than an older teen. They are curious and childlike, able to view sex as more of a playful pastime than an activity of deeply intimate attachments.

Attachments, however, inevitably form, and with them come emotional problems. A teen is likely to form an intimate bond with her first sexual partner, but of course, the bond almost always breaks. The teen, naturally enough, becomes emotionally wounded from the break and begins to close herself off from intimacy. When she eventually goes on to find another sex partner, the new bond that forms isn't as deep, but eventually breaks like the first, and the cycle continues. Each time this happens, the teen walls herself off a little more, until at last she has very little left emotionally to offer her partner. Unfortunately, these walls are not selective for particular kinds of relationships. They don't stop some bonds from forming while allowing others. A wall is a wall. A teen may turn off not only to sexual relationships, but to those of love, friendship, or trust as well.

Teens who engage in group sex may experience the same sort of emotional shutdown in a more dramatic way. Because the sexual experience is by its nature a deeply intimate and private one, teens who engage in sex in a public and nonintimate manner may actually dissociate from the act while doing it. Emotionally, they "check out" or simply go numb to get through the experience, much like a person who is going through a severe trauma. This is a natural psychological survival mechanism, which enables humans to survive emotionally overwhelming situations. It's almost as if a part of the mind, or psyche, temporarily dies, then comes back to life after the event.

This business of going numb can have serious psychological consequences for our kids. When the teen matures and feels emotionally able to handle what happened during group sex, he may actually feel traumatized. He may relive the experience on a deeper emotional level and feel intense anxiety, shame, victimization, sadness, grief, or a multitude of other emotions. In short, the part of him that pretended sex was a public event deeply hurt the part of him that knew it was meant to be private.

Aside from the psychological pain wrought from multiple partners, let's think about disease exposure. Let's say a 14-year-old girl is bisexual and has frequented lesbian "parties." Let's conservatively estimate that she had two male partners and two female partners. Let's also assume that her partners were just like her. When she swapped body fluids with her partners, how many others had she come in contact with? Fifteen. She thought that she had sex with four, but she forgot that she also "had sex" with everyone they had contacted sexually. If her partner count had jumped to seven (which is not uncommon for teens who have group sex), her contacts would have soared to 127. That means, with just those seven partners she would have come into contact with the diseases of 127 other teens. Now, statistically speaking, at least one of those 127 teens had some STD to spread around. Group sex is no joke.

CAN I WATCH? VOYEURISM

Our small town of 50,000 recently experienced an episode in which very young teenagers, ages 12 and 13, were caught having oral sex at school. Girls were performing oral sex on boys while other students watched. The boys challenged the girls as a dare. Dares have been around for a long time, haven't they? What 12-year-old can resist a dare? And a girl needs to prove that she's cool, too. She's tough, above embarrassment. But when did our culture make toughness the standard for a sexual relationship? And while performing these acts to impress other people with their coolness, whose respect did these girls gain? The boys'? Their own? How will any one of these girls feel when she returns to school in 20 years for a class reunion and sees the same faces that were in that crowd?

In another situation, a high school teacher told me how she overheard some male students talking about a party they'd attended the weekend before, where they pooled their money and paid several girls to "make out" with each other so they could watch. As the teacher listened, the boys laughed as they talked about what the girls looked like as they kissed one another, their mouths wide open, tongues entangled. Their tone was one of titillation and disgust. I wonder if they realize that what they did was prostitute these girls?

"Sexual freedom" victimizes our teens on many levels. These boys might have otherwise been pretty good kids. But living in a culture that saturates them with sexual imagery and trains them to be sexually irresponsible also teaches them to view and treat people more like objects than human beings. Their respect for others deteriorates and ultimately their respect for themselves plummets. Teen girls become nothing more than the playthings of the male libido. And teen boys are regarded as sexually demanding machines without intellects, feelings, or any emotional depth.

In the end, unrestrained sexual freedom pits our boys and girls against each other. They are not sexual partners, they are competitors and at times enemies. Each group vies to see who can more easily manipulate the other. Girls are exploited and wounded and boys get stuck in a role that drives them from one destructive, meaningless, and risky episode to the next. Of course, this doesn't happen to all teens, but it happens to thousands too many.

In the end, however, the bacteria and viruses of STDs don't care what drives kids to come together sexually. They don't care if the kids enjoy what they're doing or if psychological trauma is the result. They don't care who's watching, and they don't care if the only thing that brought skin into contact with skin was a dare. Germs have a simple purpose: to survive, multiply, and spread. Voyeurism is their ally.

EVERYTHING BUT SEX...

Teens are smart when it comes to figuring out how not to break the rules but how to come as close as possible. The "rules" when it comes to sex are maintaining your virginity and not getting pregnant or sick. So in addition to oral sex, they've integrated mutual masturbation, outercourse, and anal sex into their sexual repertoire.

Mutual masturbation involves teens who fondle one another's genitalia, sometimes to the point of orgasm, sometimes not. It can range anywhere from soft petting to aggressive, full masturbation. Mutual masturbation may seem like a "safe" way for kids to have sex, but any time body fluids are exchanged, there's a risk of disease.

Outercourse, another form of supposedly safe sex, is similar to mutual masturbation and, in fact, may include it. It usually involves intense rubbing of the genitalia against a partner's body with clothes on or off, sometimes resulting in orgasm. Often a teenage boy will ejaculate near his partner's vagina but outside of it, perhaps on her stomach or thigh.

These two techniques might sound safe enough—after all, at least they're not having actual intercourse. But any time genitalia come in contact with another person—whether it's that person's hands, mouth, or body—there is the potential for transmission of an STD. And one form of seemingly safe sexual behavior can lead very easily to a less safe form. Outercourse, for example, often leads to intercourse.

Teens who are in a relationship with a boyfriend or girlfriend and fear pregnancy will experiment with ways to sexually satisfy each other. They will start one activity, such as mutual masturbation or outercourse, but when their arousal takes over, they switch to another—often intercourse. Let's face it, once kids hit the intensity of mutual masturbation or outercourse, trying to turn back from real intercourse is like trying to throw a car into reverse while it's going 70 miles an hour down the freeway.

A DANGEROUS MIXTURE: SEX, DRUGS, AND ALCOHOL

When you mix alcohol and drugs with sexually active teenagers, you wind up with a potentially explosive and extremely risky combination. And the three are mixed together far too often. One large study conducted by the Kaiser Family Foundation found that almost one-quarter (23%) of sexually active teens and young adults—about 5.6 million nationally—report having unprotected sex because they were drinking or using drugs at the time. In that study, half of 15- to 24-year-olds said "people their age" mix alcohol or drugs and sex "a lot," and 73% believed their peers often don't use condoms when alcohol and drugs are in the picture.[17]

When adolescents drink, they lose all inhibition. To make matters worse, alcohol acts to facilitate sexual arousal in teens. While girls simply become sexually aroused, boys may also become more aggressive.

Jared's Story

When Jared was 17, he went to a friend's house one night for a party. He really didn't want to go, but a couple of his buddies would be there and he didn't want them to give him a hard time on Monday at school for not showing up. When he arrived, there were cars on the lawn and kids in the garage, halls, bedrooms, and everywhere else—about 250 teens in all. The parents who owned the house were out of town and had left their young son in charge.

When Jared walked inside, kids were trashing the furniture. They were spilling beer on the chairs, carpet, everywhere. One kid was throwing up in the living room. Jared felt disgusted and was about to leave, when he spotted this "gorgeous" girl. He was so taken with her that he felt unusually self-conscious. It took him half an hour before he got up the nerve to talk to her. What did he do to get up his nerve? He started drinking beer. It helped. He relaxed and started talking freely to everyone. By the time he introduced himself to her, he was feeling pretty lightheaded.

Before he knew it, the two of them were upstairs in a bedroom ripping each other's clothes off. There, in the home of someone he didn't really know, with a girl he'd met an hour or two earlier, Jared had intercourse. Three or four beers blurred the entire event. I could see as he talked that the episode still bothered him. The worst, Jared said, was that the next day, all he could think about was how his girlfriend, Alicia, would feel if she found out. Jared and she had been together happily for a year now. He told me that going to the party was one of the most idiotic things he'd ever done. He immensely regretted having sex with the girl and decided to tell Alicia before someone else told her. I told him that his confession took a lot of guts and I applauded him for doing so. Apparently Alicia didn't. She severed their relationship.

After that, Jared swore off alcohol. "It just made me make a terrible mistake," he said, "and I know I never would have done that if I hadn't been drinking. No more. It's not worth it."

There is another risk when drugs and alcohol influence sexual behavior: sexual abuse against teenage girls skyrockets.

Take my patient Mindy. When she was 17, Mindy went out with her boyfriend of six months. They liked going to a nearby park and smoking marijuana or drinking beer. One night, they drank and got high until about 1 A.M., then went for a walk together. After that, Mindy said, they fought. The next thing she remembered she was waking alone in the cold, damp field. Her shirt was torn and her blue jeans gone. Her legs hurt and she saw bruises developing. She walked home, took a long shower, and cried hysterically.

I first saw her a week after the incident. She was still visibly upset, and I began caring for her as a rape victim. Yes, she had been raped. Was it the fault of alcohol? No, it was her boyfriend's fault. But the alcohol and drugs certainly contributed to it. They lowered her boyfriend's inhibitions, her own judgments of safety, and any ability she had to defend herself in a horrible situation.

The Alcohol-Disease Connection

Sadly, teens drink frequently before, during, and after sex—sometimes to prepare them for it, sometimes to blot it out. Teens who are frightened, embarrassed, or hesitant in any way will drink to gain courage. They may want to be liked and accepted by peers, so they drink because this will make them feel accepted. And drinking will help them have sex—of all stripes.

Studies show that adolescents who drink engage in high-risk sexual behaviors, and HIV-related sexual behaviors. This makes sense. Teens who get drunk, or even just a little high, lose their inhibitions and try riskier sexual acts. They might toss a condom aside, have rougher sex, or try anal sex—things they would never do if they weren't drinking.

Some teens, like Mindy, drink because they need to alter their mood. Home life is hard. They feel rejected by friends. Their grades are poor and they've had one too many arguments with mom or dad. Life feels intolerable and there's no place to go, no getting free from hopelessness or sadness, so they drink. As the buzz of alcohol moves through their brain, they become vulnerable to sexual excitement. And since alcohol permits the "yes" to fall freely from their lips, they have intercourse, oral sex, and other experimentations.

But after the alcohol wears off, their mood becomes more depressed than before (because alcohol has depressant effects), and they feel worse. They numbed themselves to avoid the pain of life and now it's back in greater force because something happened the night before. Something that was supposed to be good turned out to be bad. And all of life feels worse than it did before. The way out? Drink again. Try sex again, perhaps it will be better this time. And so the cycle continues.

CYBERSEX

The two most common reasons people turn to the Internet are for health information and pornography. Among our teenagers, relatively easy access to sexually explicit information online has resulted in a plethora of kids hopping aboard the cybersex train.

They hang out in chat rooms and talk about what it feels like to have oral sex, intercourse, and anal sex, using language that would make their parents' hair stand on end. They exchange pictures and describe in graphic detail what they want to do to one another.

One reason teens like the Internet is that they can be whoever they want. A 12-year-old boy can log in as an 18-year-old girl, or a 13-year-old nerd can create an online persona of a bulked-up 25-year-old football player. But it works both ways. A 35-year-old pedophile can also log in as a 17-year-old boy and prey on unsuspecting kids. In May 2002, a 13-year-old sixth-grader in a Catholic school who made good grades, led the cheerleading squad, and was an altar girl, but who used provocative screen names and routinely had sex with partners she met in online chat rooms, was strangled to death by a married restaurant worker she met on the Internet.[18] In June 2002, a Massachusetts high school science teacher pleaded guilty for directing a 15-year-old California girl to his private Web site for a two-and-a-half-hour "cybersex" encounter.[19] In 2000, a New York engineer was sentenced to a year in jail for molesting a 15-year-old girl with whom he earlier had conducted a two-week cybersex relationship.

I recently interviewed Claudia Bennett, a professor at Eastern Michigan University who teaches a college course on media and its effects on teenagers. She described to me the explosion of teen sex through Internet chat rooms. She told me of teens who chat online about what they want to do sexually to one another in graphic detail, then go to school the next day, sit in the same classroom, and never speak to each other. This is a peculiar psychological phenomenon. It's almost as if the participants "compartmentalize themselves." In other words, they have divided themselves into private portions, public portions, and other portions reserved only for specific groups. When they go online, they share parts of themselves that they would never share face to face.

What is so disturbing about teen cybersex, however, is that private information is often shared publicly and in a detached manner. If teens who have group sex become desensitized to forming intimate bonds, teens who have cybersex avoid emotional bonds altogether. In a sense, they're actually training themselves to *not* bond during sex. This can have serious consequences as they mature and can cause them to have very real difficulty forming meaningful intimate relationships down the road.

Ms. Bennett, like many teachers I have spoken with, sounded disheartened as she described the situation. "Internet sex," she said, "has become part of the kids' lives. I used to ask my students what impact the Internet had on their lives and they looked at me confused. They didn't understand what I was asking because the Internet is part of them. It's like their arm or their leg. They can't imagine life without it. It is simply integrated into them. But what about these young kids now? Cybersex is shaping their sex lives. Twelve- and 13-year-old teens are having cybersex before they have real sex. It is shaping their expectations, it changes their relationships. It will even begin shaping their sexuality. What will happen when it [cybersex] becomes as integrated into the younger kids' lives the way the larger Internet has become integrated into the lives of my [college] students?"

I fear that for many students, it already has. If you have any doubts about whether your teen logs into chat rooms and has cybersex, you'd better find out. Ms. Bennett encouraged her students to ask their younger siblings if they were involved. She said that her students (19- and 20-year-olds) were shocked to hear what their 13-, 14-, and 15-year-old siblings revealed to them. Yes, they said that "everyone" had cybersex. It was just another thing to do and no one wanted to be left out. If her college-age students were left in the dark about their siblings' Internet exploits, how much more in the dark are we?

GOOD SEX/BAD SEX

As I've lectured about teen sex around the country, I've noticed two assumptions commonly made by people who disagree with my stance on teenage sex. Those who think that teenage sexual activity is healthy and good assume that because I encourage teens to practice self-control, to hold off on sexual activity until they are in a committed, monogamous relationship, that I am a sex-hater. They assume that when I encourage teens to erect boundaries around their sexuality and hold off so they can experience true lovemaking in the future, rather than just sex for sex' sake, I do so because I think sex is bad, unpleasant, or shameful. They couldn't be more wrong.

It is precisely because I respect sexual activity so highly that I encourage my teenage patients to do the same. I want nothing more for them than that they ultimately experience tremendous joy and pleasure from their future sexual encounters.

The other camp I run into assumes that because I condone sexual control in teenagers, I dislike homosexuals. I find this really strange. One hostile host of a radio program asked me during an interview, "Okay, Dr. Meeker. So you say that sex is dangerous for teens. But how can you say this and take good care of gay kids? What do you tell them, *huh*?" His tone was biting, communicating to me and his listeners that being anti–teen sex meant being anti-gay.

I responded honestly to his challenge. "I tell my gay patients exactly what I tell straight kids. That sex can kill them." To me a teen is a teen. I took an oath 20 years ago to do my best to keep my patients healthy. This isn't about gay or straight, it's about all teens and all sexual activity. It's not a political issue, it's a medical issue. The best thing for teens, I firmly believe, is waiting.

The truth is, gay teen boys are at higher risk for HIV, hepatitis B, and many other STDs than straight kids and they need to know that. Being ethical is about giving truthful information that could save a person's life, and I don't think there's anything much more unethical than withholding lifesaving information.

The bottom line is simply this: I don't hate sex, I love sex. I think it's one of the most profound experiences we humans can have, regardless of orientation. The fact of the matter is, I love people. And I want them to enjoy long, healthy lives.

PART III

What To Know, What To Do

TEN

■ The average age of young girls at the onset of puberty has dropped
from 12 to 10 years.

Adolescent in Body and Mind

ADOLESCENCE IS A TIME OF TIDAL changes in the bodies of boys and
girls. Everything is different, from their height and weight to the
timbre of their voices. Hormones give them strange, new, powerful
feelings, and the people around them begin to treat them as young
adults. While their bodies develop, so do their minds, and both are
driven by and must adjust to all these changes. When I first thought
about approaching these subjects—body and mind—I planned to
write about them separately, but it soon became apparent that I
couldn't, because they are not separate. They weave together intimately into the wonderful, delightful, and mysterious fabric of our
sons and daughters at this time in their lives. We need to understand
this profoundly, if we are to help them avoid becoming victims of the
epidemic that has affected so many young people already.

WHEN PUBERTY STRIKES

Something happened to a patient of mine, a young girl named Andrea, that may strike you as unusual. Andrea entered puberty when she was 7 years old.

Something fundamental has changed in the biology of human female development over the past couple of decades: The average age of young girls at the onset of puberty has dropped from 12 to 10 years. Physicians aren't exactly sure why, but some speculate that improved nutrition plays a role, while others wonder about the effects of food additives, and still others point the finger at environmental factors. We don't yet have any answers. Unfortunately, we do have a new set of problems. How could we not, with little girls becoming women practically overnight?

Andrea's Story

Andrea's mother first discovered that something was happening when Andrea complained she didn't want to go to school anymore because her friends kept saying she smelled funny. Mom had a simple solution: she bought her daughter some deodorant. But a few months later, Andrea's breasts began to develop, and pubic hair followed. At that point she came to see me. Warning bells went off in my head. Better make doubly sure nothing is wrong, I told myself, so I performed a multitude of blood tests, an ultrasound of her abdomen, and even considered getting an MRI of her head to check for tumors. All of her tests failed to turn up any abnormalities other than what we call benign precocious puberty. Although I needed to rule out any possible medical condition, that was actually the result I had expected. While it's true that Andrea's situation was unusual, it was only slightly so. If she had been just one year older, she would have fallen well within the norm.

Andrea started having her period before she entered the second grade. I offered to write a prescription for medication that would stop her menstruating, but her mother decided against it. Interfering medically with a child's natural growth and development could be a tricky and dangerous business. So instead Andrea had to carry Kotex in her backpack. One day, a few spilled out and a couple of classmates saw them. It was all the bait the young kids needed. They began whispering about her and calling her a freak. By the third grade, Andrea found it difficult to hide her breasts beneath her shirt. She had to wear a bra. Not the cut-off-undershirt kind. A real bra.

Girls entering puberty early often face terrible teasing from their classmates, who can be brutal on a child with breasts, body odor, or underarm hair. A young girl who menstruates will often be stigmatized by her peers, and any child who needs to wear a bra at age 9 or 10 will often run into spiteful jealousy among her friends. All of this happened to Andrea.

As her mother and I tried to guide Andrea through those tough, early years, here's what I saw: She hated school—kids were still calling her a freak. Her grades dropped and she became irritable at home and in class. She actually showed signs of depression. By the time she had reached the fourth grade, boys had already begun identifying her as a "sex fiend." She didn't like this, of course, but she didn't know how to respond. She wasn't even sure what kids were talking about. She didn't know what sex was.

Early puberty often creates these dilemmas for young girls. Budding breasts, pubic hair, and menstruation attract attention and can force a girl to confront her sexuality before she's psychologically ready. Emotionally she may still want to play with dolls and collect stuffed animals, but at the same time she's choosing from 20 different deodorant brands and using sanitary pads or tampons. No wonder she's confused! She may feel overwhelmed by her changing body. She sees that she's beginning to look like mom, but she doesn't want to look like mom. She wants to be a kid and let mom be the adult.

In Andrea's case, dealing with sexual issues before she was ready proved traumatic. We finally ended up sending her to a counselor in the fifth grade because she became more depressed, and in response to the boys' taunting, her behavior started to become sexualized. She was flirting—both with the boys and with disaster. But this wasn't the kind of flirting you would expect from a child of her age. She wasn't teasing the boys to get them to chase her around the playground. She was enticing them by asking them if they wanted to see her private areas. Fortunately, her mother and an astute teacher caught wind of these episodes and intervened before Andrea was actually able to follow through.

How could a girl who so hated sexual teasing suddenly become so sexual? Premature puberty had thrust her into an adult world that she wasn't ready for emotionally. Not only did she have to contend with her own feelings, but she was forced to contend with the feelings and reactions of the kids around her. She couldn't stop the teasing, but teasing was better than getting no attention at all. And if her body could get her more attention. . . . Well, why not? Unfortunately, this strategy—unconscious on her part—got Andrea into trouble and ultimately made her feel even more like a freak, worse about herself, and in need of counseling.

What if Andrea's mom hadn't been observant enough to recognize that her daughter was having trouble? Suppose Andrea kept maturing and made it to junior high without any intervention? Now she's 12, has periods regularly, and her breasts look like those of an 18-year-old. Instead of third-grade boys, she has 13-, 14-, and 15-year-old classmates asking her for a "peek at her privates." What would she do if no one had stepped in to help her earlier? Would she please her classmates to get attention? Would she have sex?

As Andrea's story illustrates, there's little doubt that early puberty sets girls up for early sexual encounters. With so many girls now entering puberty by age 8 or 9, and the risk for disease rising so dramatically among kids who have sex at a very young age, we might see the STD epidemic grow far worse.

What can we do about it? For one thing, we can be there for our daughters. We can try to understand what they're going through and give them whatever help they need to make their way through the minefield of experiencing childhood in an adultlike body. We can become active and try to change the world they live in, which seems all too ready to sexualize little girls in films, television, and magazines. And we can simply remember who they are. However mature a young girl's body may look, we need to remind ourselves that a child lives inside. Finally, we must be ready to intervene strongly if we discover our daughters are becoming sexual long before it's appropriate.

STDS AND THE ADOLESCENT GIRL'S BODY

One of the strongest reasons to encourage your daughters to wait as long as they can before becoming sexually active is that their bodies are not ready for it, even though they may think otherwise. A young girl's cervix (opening to the uterus) develops slowly, and has several physiological differences from that of an older woman. These differences put a young girl at higher risk for STDs.

To the naked eye, a cervix looks like a plump doughnut with a tiny hole in the center. In young girls, tall, narrow, reddish-pink cells cover the cervix. These cells, called columnar cells, form a layer of skin called the ectropion. The pinkness comes from the rich blood supply in the columnar cells, which provides a wonderful medium for bacteria and viruses.

On the outer edge of the cervix are flatter, tougher cells, called squamous cells, which have a more "smushed" appearance than the columnar cells. After childbirth, or by the time a woman reaches her mid-20s, these tougher squamous cells move into the center of the cervix, replacing the reddish ectropion layer and columnar cells and, in the process, better protecting the cervix. Because they don't have the same rich blood supply as the columnar cells, squamous cells are less attractive to the viruses and bacteria that cause sexually transmitted diseases.

In the adolescent female, a specific type of cell lining the inside of the cervical canal extends onto the outer surface of the cervix, where exposure to sexually transmitted pathogens is greater. These cells are more vulnerable to infections such as chlamydia and gonorrhea. As women age, this vulnerable tissue recedes and usually no longer extends onto the outer surface of the cervix.

Then there is the difference in the cervical tissue of a 15-year-old versus an older woman. Just as a teenager's skin and the skin of a 30-year-old woman are different, so too is cervical tissue. In a young girl, this tissue is softer, more easily permeated by viruses and bacteria. In an older woman, it's tougher, harder, and thus able to better ward off bacteria, viruses, and other pathogens.

In addition, the cervical mucus, which serves a protective role, differs in teenagers and older women. Many girls will menstruate without ovulating for the first year or two. When this happens, the mucus in their cervix is thinner, and has a more liquid consistency that, for some unknown reason, is more attractive for viruses and bacteria, providing a richer environment for growth than an older woman's cervical mucus.

The attractiveness of a young girl's cervix to bacteria and virus infections seems to lead, for some unknown reason, to a much greater risk for pelvic inflammatory disease than that experienced by adult women. Overall, an adolescent with chlamydia or gonorrhea has a one in eight chance of developing PID, compared with a 30-year-old with the same infection, who has a one in eighty chance.

Your teenage daughter needs you to help her realize that her body isn't ready to handle physically what yours or mine can. Tell her. Talk to her and help her to wait for much better sex—great sex—when she is older. When her chances of getting PID, even if she does happen to get chlamydia or gonorrhea, drop to one in eighty. Don't let her become one of the one in eight.

WHEN BOYS REACH PUBERTY

Boys begin moving through puberty between the ages of 12 and 16. (Unlike with girls, we haven't seen puberty start any earlier in boys.)

As levels of testosterone rise in boys, their penis grows longer, their testicles grow bigger, and they grow body and pubic hair. Soon, facial hair appears and their voice changes. They become sexually aroused and often experience their first wet dreams and regular erections. After puberty is well under way, a growth spurt occurs.

My personal experience has led me to believe that puberty can be harder for boys than for girls. There are several reasons for this. First, many boys are hesitant to discuss how they feel about the changes they are experiencing. As they see facial hair erupt and experience their first wet dreams, for instance, some feel ambivalent about growing up. Their bodies march ahead into manhood, but their emotions hang back. Or they may simply be confused about what is happening to them. But all too often, they're left to cope with these problems on their own, because "guys just don't talk about that stuff." With no guidance, it's easy for a boy to follow the lead of the media and his peers in defining his own sense of manhood. Unfortunately, these aren't dependable guides, and they can lead a boy into unsafe places, as we'll see in a moment.

Aside from feeling hesitant to express confusion or stresses about puberty, many teen boys also face intense pressure to become sexually active. Their culture equates masculinity with sexual activity—particularly frequent and varied sexual activity—before they have a chance to figure out for themselves what being masculine means to them personally. Let me explain how this happens.

As puberty occurs in a teen boy, he watches himself. Are his arms getting more muscular? How dense is his beard? And then he watches his buddies. How are their beards? Any hair on their legs yet? He hears stories about sex they have with girls and wonders what it feels like. He hears about putting condoms on the right way and the wrong way and wonders whether it just might be safer to try oral sex first and skip the whole condom thing. He feels the excitement of sexual arousal, which may be overwhelming at times. What does he do with those urges? He hears his buddies talk about having sex with a lot of other girls and having it a lot of different ways (oral sex, etc.). He sees men (usually young and single) having sex with women on TV and in movies and sees sex plastered across the covers of men's magazines. In his mind, he makes a leap between his sexual urges and what he should do about them. He decides, maybe unconsciously, that he should have a lot of sex because that's what he sees guys all around him do and because you have to have sex to be a "real man." So he tries it. He tries once, then twice, and then again and again.

The pressures of coping with tremendous sexual urges, trying to appear manly among peers, and being hesitant to discuss their feelings about puberty can make teen boys incredibly vulnerable to having sex at a young age and with numerous partners. And both of these, in an age of an STD epidemic, spell disaster for our boys.

So here's how we can help. First, let your kids know that being a man is a good thing. It is not something that they need to be frightened about. Let your son know that he will be a man in his own unique way. He has the freedom to be different from any bad role models he has seen.

Help him identify pressures he faces because he is going through puberty. Show him specifically where those messages are coming from—magazines, movies, etc. Believe it or not, you can do this in a way that doesn't make you look like a movie-hating, sex-hating parent. Ask what messages he's getting and what he thinks about them. Let him know that you are his advocate in helping him define what being a man is all about for him and that you want to make sure that the "real" him isn't suffocated by messages about being male that he bumps into daily. (Teens love having advocates.) Teach him that all healthy boys become sexually excited by things they see. So, tell him to recognize when his happens and let him know that just because he gets excited when a girl walks by in a tight top, he doesn't need to act on that feeling. It will pass. When he realizes that his feelings are normal and that someone understands, he feels less frightened of them and more importantly he feels that he can control them, they needn't control him. This brings boys tremendous relief.

Acknowledge that his emotional and physical feelings will be intense and that's okay. They're supposed to be. You don't have to tell him specifics about masturbation, but if you tell him in a straightforward, simple manner that boys commonly release their sexual feelings privately, he'll know what you mean and feel less guilty. Many boys feel guilty about masturbating and regardless of a parent's moral or ethical feelings about it, the truth is, boys experience it during puberty.

Regarding other physiological changes puberty brings to boys, simply stay attuned to those changes and be proactive when you think it appropriate. If your son breaks out with acne, don't wait for him to ask for help. Take him to a doctor and get it cleared up. His face is every bit as important to his self-esteem as a girl's is to her. Buy him shaving cream and a razor when he needs it (or a little before) and make a fuss over it. This lets him know that you like the changes you see and you like him becoming a man. If he needs deodorant, buy it without his asking and put it in his bathroom next to his toothbrush. Simply being on the lookout for physical changes that you see happening and acknowledging those changes in a positive, respectful way will ease the stresses he may feel and most importantly, lets him know that you like them.

A final word of caution: When a boy reaches puberty, many of us make remarks that we perceive as harmless but in fact can hurt him. Saying things like, "Boy, you can certainly catch any girl you want now" can be tough on boys. What you meant to say is that he is attractive and should feel good about himself. But what he may have heard was that he is sexual and should be able to sleep with anyone he wants. So be careful.

SEX AND SEXUALITY

When boys and girls hit puberty, it's like a bomb goes off in their bodies and their minds, leaving them with new feelings, ideas, and opinions. One part of these normal psychological and cognitive changes is the blossoming of their sexuality.

Don't confuse sexuality with sexual activity. The two are related, but different. A teenager's sexuality is that part of her character that prepares her for sexual activity, as well as deeper relationships involving love, intimacy, and respect. It's a critical part of a teenager's identity, and influences her ability to relate to others.

Sexual activity, on the other hand, is the act of having sex.

Unfortunately, many teens *do* confuse sexuality with sexual activity. When teens begin to mature sexually, they feel confused about what to do with the strong, unfamiliar sexual feelings washing over them. Boys begin trying to define their own masculinity, comparing it to other boys around them and wondering if they "measure up." Too often, however, they define masculinity as sexuality. Girls begin to fantasize about romance, and use clothing, makeup, and perfume to define their own femininity. And, too often, these accoutrements become tools to attract the opposite sex, to feel "sexy," to lead to sex.

Take my patient Caleb. At 16, he came to me for a regular physical and immunizations. As I worked my way down my list of questions, I asked about girlfriends. "Oh, yeah," he replied. "Lots of them." As he described his relationships, I learned that they were really just frequent sexual encounters with girls his age or younger (even 13 or 14) whom he barely knew. Basically, he was sleeping around indiscriminately—something he told me he enjoyed. And, no surprise, upon examination I found he was infected with chlamydia, which he'd surely spread to many of those young girls.

As we talked more, it soon became clear why he behaved this way. When he was 3 years old, his father left the family, and had had numerous sexual relationships since. So there was no one to show Caleb the difference between feelings of sexuality and sexual activity. Instead, he just mimicked what he saw his father doing. And, since he admired his father, he figured that having numerous sexual encounters was the best way to embrace his own masculinity and sexuality. Thus, Caleb learned to define his sexuality by the number of girls he slept with. He never learned to develop other masculine strengths that lead to respectful and romantic intimate relationships with women.

Caleb is not alone. Many of our teenage boys are taught that being sexual means being sexually active, whether they're taught by a parent, or by the music they listen to, the movies they see, and the magazines they read.

Just as their sexuality begins to bloom, teenagers also experience three major psychological developments that are tightly entwined with their developing sexuality: emancipation, identity formation, and the slow and gradual development of abstract thinking. Let's take a look at each one in turn.

Emancipation

An important part of adolescence is separating from one's parents, in a process called emancipation. Teens usually embark upon this around puberty, beginning with baby steps (driving, getting a job, developing their own opinions) and ending with the giant leap into college or on to other adult endeavors.

Although teens *want* to separate from you, the process itself is frightening for them. That's why you often see your teenager taking one step forward and two steps back. Your 15-year-old daughter might be into giggling about boys and trying new makeup, while at the same time she sleeps with her stuffed animal from childhood and still wants a goodnight kiss from you.

During this process, teenagers start redefining their emotional relationship with you, moving from that of parent and child to that of parent and adult. At the same time, they're separating from you physically. Suddenly, it seems they're never home. They may refuse to go on family vacations, or even to go out to dinner as a family. They walk apart from you when you're in public places, and head straight to their room when they get home. Some get after-school jobs that keep them out of the house, or start spending inordinate amounts of time at a friend's house, perhaps even "adopting" that other family as their own.

They're not doing this to abandon you, but to redefine their relationship with you, to move from a posture of physical dependence to physical independence. It's a tough transition for both parent and adolescent, and, luckily, it occurs gradually, or none of us would survive it!

Emancipation takes many forms. Some teens deliberately do things they know will annoy their parents, such as skipping chores, breaking curfew, or talking back. They're not doing these things *just* to be obnoxious (although it often seems that way) but, subconsciously, as a way to tear themselves away from you. This testing of the rules is their way of saying that things are changing. And with those changes, they want fewer restrictions and redefined boundaries. They want to be seen as an emerging adult, not as a child. This doesn't mean they don't want *any* rules, as we'll see later.

This testing is similar to the way a toddler tests boundaries. He'll wander off just a bit from you to see what happens—always keeping you within his sight. Teenagers do the same thing. When they break curfew, they're really saying: "How far can I go?"

When teens exhibit these "testing" behaviors, of course, we get angry. That anger puts another barrier between parent and teen, enhancing that feeling of separation. In a teenager's mind, it's easier to need a person less if you're mad at them. Sometimes they even pick a fight so they can feel mad, and thus have a good reason to move away from you.

For instance, I overheard the following exchange between Bo, 13, and his mother. "I decided to go out with my friends tonight and I'll be home around eleven-thirty," Bo told his mother.

"Eleven-thirty! I don't think so! Your curfew is 10 P.M.," his mother said, shocked and angry.

"So what? It should be changed. What do you think I'm going to do? Don't you trust me?" Bo demanded.

A huge fight ensued between the two, ending with Bo storming into his room and his mother in tears.

Bo's assertion of his new sense of independence is typical of early adolescence. He deliberately picked a fight with his mother so he could have an arena in which to begin negotiating his independence and separation. Of course, he doesn't recognize that he did this, for, as you'll see below, he still lacks the sophisticated reasoning that would enable him to see the full scope and consequences of his actions.

Teenagers turn to sex for the same reasons. Sex makes them feel more grown up, more like an adult. It provides a sense of independence and freedom from parental authority. It's a behavior parents can't see or control, an action in which the teenager is the one in control, the one making the decisions. This provides an incredible sense of power, and provides yet another way for the teenager to physically and emotionally separate from his parents.

The challenge for parents is to find safer ways for teenagers to exert their independence, like finding a first job, opening their own checking account, taking responsibility for a car. You can provide "safer" freedoms—the freedom to choose their own clothes, hairstyles, the way they decorate their room. Helping them find safer ways to define their independence, while maintaining certain boundaries, will reduce the risk that they'll turn to sex for that independence.

The balance between providing more freedom without totally relinquishing all rules is tricky. If you're too rigid, and don't give your teen *some* opportunities for independence, they'll rebel and look for them on their own, often turning to the risky behaviors of sex, drinking, and drugs.

But if you give them too much freedom, they may feel as if they've been prematurely thrust out of the nest, maybe because you don't love them. Many parents of our generation give too much freedom too soon to our kids because we want to teach them autonomy. While your intentions may be rooted in love, your teen feels just the opposite—that he is unloved. Remember, *rules and boundaries make teens feel loved.* Parents who abandon too many rules too quickly communicate to their kids that the teens are adult enough to make all their own decisions. Thus, teens begin acting in "adult" ways. To them, this means drinking, doing drugs, and having sex.

I often see this in my own practice. Many concerned parents give their teens too much freedom too soon, not because they don't love their kids, but because they're anxious to prove their trust. Teens don't understand this; they just haven't developed the kind of complex thinking required to comprehend this kind of action. So they get confused and angry. They look for love and a sense of belonging wherever they can—sometimes in sex.

That's what happened with Myra. As soon as I saw her and her parents in my office, I knew it was serious. I could hear them fighting even before I entered the exam room.

"I just don't know what to do with her!" her dad blurted out before I even sat down. "She's out of control." Ever since Myra turned 14, she'd been very restless and her parents had adopted a hands-off approach. When Myra wanted to go to parties with older kids, her parents let her. When she wanted to date a boy who was 18, they let her. The consequences were predictable: Myra got pregnant and had an abortion—an event her parents didn't learn about until several months after the fact. After the abortion, Myra became sullen and irritable. She hated being home, she wanted to be out as much as possible. So her parents let her. The more she pulled away, the more her parents let go, afraid that if they cracked down and set limits, she'd only get into more trouble.

What prompted this particular visit? I asked. Myra didn't answer. "She thinks she might be pregnant again," her mother said. As her father and mother spoke I could see a coldness in Myra's eyes. Her body language was stiff and angry. She looked like she wanted to scream and cry at the same time.

When we finished talking, I examined Myra. Fortunately, she wasn't pregnant. But she did have gonorrhea. Although I treated Myra for the STD, I urged her and her parents to see a good family counselor. At first, her parents didn't want to go because they felt embarrassed. They insisted they loved her intensely and had always worked hard to be good parents. But they made one huge mistake. They gave Myra too much freedom before she could handle it.

As Myra herself said: "At first, I liked the independence. But later, I wished they'd given me a curfew, like the other kids had. I wanted the rules back." She was desperately searching for proof that someone loved her and cared—just small things, like her dad waiting up for her to make sure she was okay. After a while, thinking her parents didn't care about her all, she began having sex, hoping, deep down, she said, that she would get caught.

Myra got her wish and, with help from a good counselor, began to feel the love her parents had for her. Once her parents realized they could better communicate their love for her by providing boundaries and rules, Myra quickly settled down and stopped having sex to get their attention.

One final word of caution about emancipation: When your teen breaks those non-negotiable rules (and feisty teens will break them to test your reaction), you must enforce serious consequences. I recommend that non-negotiable rules center around safety and respect for others. For instance, driving and drinking can kill, so this is a good, non-negotiable rule. In our house, one of our own non-negotiable rules with our children centers around driving. They can't speed. If they get a speeding ticket, the car gets taken away for a predetermined period of time, say three to six months, depending on their age. These rules and enforced consequences are critical to our teens. Just like the laws of your town, state, and country, they work to keep a collective society civilized. The family is the first place teenagers learn how rules and consequences work.

Identity Formation

As kids seek emancipation from parental control, they're also trying to figure out just who they are. I frequently ask teens to describe themselves to me. Since most kids love to talk about themselves they dive into a list that typically goes like this: "I'm pretty good at soccer, my grades are okay, and I like clothes." But if I ask them to describe themselves as their best friend sees them, the list of attributes is quite different. "Well, she'd say I'm a really good listener, I try to be a really good friend. Sometimes we get into arguments but I'm the first one that tries to patch things up. She might say I help her a lot and I'm always there for her."

This is the inner and outer identity, and it is during the teenage years that adolescents are struggling to define these two sides of the same coin.

The outer self is what they look like and how they behave. They spend a lot of time trying to improve this outer self, trying to fit in with their peers in the way they dress, wear their hair, even the way they walk or talk. Included in this outer self are all the things teenagers *do*. The sports they play, their actions at parties, the grades they get in class. They work to excel in these areas not only because it makes them feel good about themselves, but to gain greater acceptance from others.

The inner self they describe is "the real me." The person with the deep feelings and secret thoughts. This is the part of themselves teenagers share only with those with whom they are closest. Frequently they lament, "No one understands the 'real' me." This inner self is harder to know than the outer self, because its qualities are more intangible. But it begins with qualities of character. Things such as compassion, good listening, personal opinions, and values. It is here, in this "inner self," that the real grappling takes place. Here that a teen wonders about and worries about life after adolescence. About true likes and dislikes. Here that the fears about growing up, about friendships, about abilities, really live.

As teens work to form both their inner and outer identities, they experiment a lot, trying on different personas in much the same way we try on shoes. They try different clothes, hairstyles, and hobbies, often venturing toward behaviors and dress designed to gain peer acceptance (and shock parents, thus, again, helping them separate). Part of this experimenting involves trying out "adult" behavior—drinking, smoking, having sex.

For even as teenagers work to learn their inner and outer identity, their sexuality is bursting. Just how does this sexuality fit into this new identity?

Boys, for instance, may believe that being sexually active makes them more masculine, more grown up, and more manly, so they try it. Girls may think it makes them more popular, more feminine, more "cool."

But this is backwards! Sex shouldn't shape a teenager's identity; *their identity and character should shape their decisions and feelings about having sex.*

Josh, 17, knew this very well. I've known Josh since he was in grade school. He's always had a close relationship with his parents, so even when puberty hit, things remained fairly steady. They struggled with the typical curfew issues, and Josh tested his parents on many occasions. A couple of times he was grounded for staying out too late when he didn't tell his parents where he was. But he enjoyed his home life, he said, and didn't really have that many complaints.

He met Julie when he was 16. They began dating seriously and talked about having sex, but decided to wait. When I asked him why, he told me about his relationship with his father. Every year, the two of them went fishing for a week. They spent the time talking about personal issues and his dad encouraged Josh to decide what *he* felt was right, then stick to his guns. He told Josh the young boy never needed to prove himself to anyone, that he was great just the way he was. Those times with his father had tremendous power in shaping Josh's feelings about his identity and his sexuality. They taught him that he was a strong person, able to make good decisions and carry them out. By spending time with him, talking and listening to him, and having fun with him, Josh's father taught his son that masculinity is about much more than sexuality, and that relationships are about much more than sex. And yet, I'll bet Josh's dad had no idea of the impact those fishing trips had on the boy.

But if a teen decides to go in the other direction and become sexually active, the decision will have a tremendous effect on that teenager's identity formation. It may change the way the teenager thinks, feels, and relates to others. It may even change his core moral values. For sexual experiences touch teens on a deeply emotional level, influencing the way they feel about themselves and others—and it's not always positive.

When Kathy was 16, she started dating Rob, also 16. They did everything together. They watched each other's basketball games, helped each other during stressful times at home and at school, were each other's best friends. He made her cookies and she sent him flowers. He even came to one of her appointments with me once because he was worried about her. Their relationship clearly influenced their own identity formation. As she told me: Rob made her "better" than she felt she could be on her own.

After about six months, they started having sex. It was a relationship of tremendous respect, and Rob always wore a condom. I was sure that these two mature kids, who seemed to have a more mature relationship than many married people I knew, would one day get married. But after a year and a half, Rob decided he needed "some space." When he broke off their relationship, Kathy was devastated. She'd adored and loved him. When he left, she said, she felt he took part of her with him.

Soon after the breakup, she began having problems concentrating and withdrew from her friends. Luckily, her parents supported her and helped her pull her life back on track. When I saw her after her first year of college, I asked how she was doing and got an answer I didn't expect.

"I hate to think about him," she said. "After he left for college, he kind of went off the deep end. He got into drugs really bad and started hanging around the wrong crowd. I can't believe it." She was still clearly hurt, both *because* of him and *for* him. "How about you?" I asked. "Any new relationships on the horizon?"

"Nope. And I don't want any. I'm haunted by him. I trusted him. He knew me better than anyone. We shared everything. We knew everything about each other. We had great sex, too. How could I have been so stupid? I don't trust myself anymore. I don't know what I want, what I believe, and what I don't believe."

It had been more than two years since the breakup, but Kathy still felt the great hurt of that early foray into sexual intimacy. Because her identity wasn't fully formed during her relationship with Rob, the experience scarred her in a permanent way, like a footprint in wet cement. Today, she has difficulty forming strong attachments, even to friends, because she's afraid to trust them and herself.

Inability to Think in the Abstract

How many times have you sat down with your teenager, told him about an important issue or event, then asked his opinion. Too often, rather than an articulate, well-thought-out response, all you get is a shrug of the shoulders followed by a mumbled, "Uhhh, I dunno." Surely this must be one of the most frustrating things about dealing with teenagers. They *look* like adults. They want—and demand—adult responsibility. So of course we expect them to *think* like adults. Big mistake.

At the beginning of puberty, teenagers simply haven't developed the kind of abstract thinking that guides most adults. They're still functioning on a concrete, black-and-white level. They have difficulty linking ideas and concepts together and understanding how one might affect another. They have problems seeing things from another person's perspective, putting themselves into another's shoes. This can, at times, make them seem as if they have no compassion. They do; they just don't know how to express it. They also have a difficult time understanding the long-term consequences of their actions. That, for instance, sex today could lead to a baby in nine months or a sexually transmitted diseases in two weeks.

I remember giving a lecture on eating disorders several years ago. My 14-year-old daughter was in the audience waiting patiently for me to finish. At the end of my lecture about why girls starve themselves, about their depression and psychological stresses, she came up to me and, in a disgusted voice, said, "Mom, I just don't get it. What's their problem? If a kid won't eat, you should just tell their parents to put them in the army, because they'll make them eat." Her concrete thought process led her to see a simple problem that required a simple solution. She simply couldn't fathom the complexity of eating disorders.

Another ramification of this concrete thinking manifests itself in the egocentricity of teenagers. Put simply, they think life revolves around them. When they need to go somewhere, they don't understand why you can't drop what you're doing and drive them. If they need a new outfit for a dance, they don't understand the fact that the car payment is due, and that there is no extra cash. This egocentricity often leads teens to act impulsively, ignoring the consequences to anyone else. Teenage boys, in particular, may struggle with the need to have their sexual desires met quickly. When they feel the physical desire to have sex, they want to do it right here, right now, regardless of the consequences or how it affects anyone else. This, of course, can be very dangerous. If teens feel entitled to have all their sexual urges met when *they* want them met, not when the time is right, they set themselves up for all the dangers of early sexual activity, primarily pregnancy, STDs, and depression.

Part of this egocentricity displays itself as a kind of "personal fable." Teenagers are certain they possess unusual abilities to endure dangers that would harm others. The personal fable says that, yes, people get hurt—but not me. That's why teenagers do such stupid things, like driving 90 miles per hour, spending days in the hot sun without sunscreen, jumping off bridges into unknown bodies of water, or having sex—protected or unprotected—with multiple partners.

Consider Jessica. She was 15 when she came to see me because, despite a poor appetite and dieting, she was gaining weight. I took a complete medical history, then left the room so she could change into a gown for the examination. When I pulled back the gown, I was shocked by her protuberant belly. I placed my hands over her swollen abdomen and felt the heels of a 7- to 8-month-old fetus kicking. The kicks were so intense, they were visible through her skin.

"Do you feel anything in your belly?" I asked.

"Yeah, a lot of gas," she said.

"Jessica," I started, "you've got a huge baby in your belly. Can you feel it move?" I don't know why I was surprised by her denial. This wasn't the first time I'd seen it in an adolescent patient.

"I *can't* be pregnant, Dr. Meeker! You're crazy! I've only had sex once and we've broke up!"

Jessica's denial was a classic example of the personal fable.

Unfortunately, we can't speed up the processes of abstract thinking and we can't zap our teens out of their own personal fable. Only time can do that. In the meantime, however, we must realize that this kind of thinking places our children at tremendous risk, and we must work with them to sidestep the temptations they're not mature enough to resist alone.

ELEVEN

■ Teens say their parents have the greatest influence on their sexual decision making; more than friends, teachers, and the media.

Connectedness

I HAVE A DEEP BELIEF THAT IS BASED neither on psychological theory nor on studies, research, and experimental data, but rather on what my heart, my intuition, tells me. My belief is this: Relationships with other people are what make our lives worth living. We need friends to talk with when we're lonely, people to care for us when we're sick, spouses or partners to love us whether we're rich or poor, fat or thin, ugly or beautiful, young or old. I believe this is true for everyone, even teens, who may seem to reject the love we offer and confound us with their antisocial behaviors and rebelliousness.

The fact is that when teens have close ties with family and friends, they are more productive, happier, and less likely to get into trouble. They develop a sense of belonging, of being part of a larger group, and feel an unspoken trust that the people who are important to them will always be there for them, no matter what the circumstance.

This unwavering sense of belonging and trust is the very substance of good relationships, and it is the strength that can keep them out of trouble or even save their lives. We have a word for it: connectedness.

OUR TEENAGERS WANT CONNECTEDNESS WITH US

In 1997, one of the most complete studies ever conducted on teenagers and high-risk behaviors was published in the *Journal of the American Medical Association*. The National Longitudinal Study of Adolescent Health (the "Add Health Study," funded by the National Institute of Child Health and Human Development and seventeen other federal agencies) set out to determine two things: What role family, friends, school, and community have in influencing teens to make healthy choices for themselves, and what role they have in encouraging unhealthy, self-destructive choices.

The fieldworkers interviewed 90,000 kids in grades seven through twelve from 145 different schools. They asked hundreds of questions and recorded thousands of answers. Then they went further, look-ing into the children's lives, studying their environment, their par-ents, and where they lived.

They found that the two most important factors in keeping teens out of trouble were a sense of connectedness with parents and like-wise with an adult figure at school, such as a teacher or counselor, who expresses care and concern for them. During a time when par-ents were repeatedly taught that peers were "everything to teens," the results of this study blew the lid off of that notion.

The authors defined parental connectedness as having a "high degree of closeness, caring, and satisfaction with parental relationships, whether resident or nonresident, mother or father, feeling understood, loved, wanted, and paid attention to by family members."

Among the factors that helped keep kids from making self-destructive or unhealthy choices such as having sex at a young age were teen/parent activities, parental presence at key times during the day (in the morning, after school, at dinner, and at bedtime), and parental expectations of high academic performance. Another important factor was the perception that parents disapproved of teenagers having sex, even with contraception.

In an age when politicians argue over sex education and educators war over condom distribution, this answer—connectedness—seems almost too simple, but my experience with my own patients has convinced me of the truth of these results. Parents and teachers who build solid relationships with teens have a far greater impact on them than do sex education programs and media messages.

Kay, the mother of one of my patients, is a good example.

Kay's son Joe was one of those kids who probably had mild attention-deficit disorder. Since early elementary school, he had always been the class clown and did whatever he needed to do to get attention from friends and teachers. Naturally, this sometimes got him into trouble.

When high school came and Joe turned 16, Kay knew that the next few years could be rough. Joe didn't like school. He liked painting and he wanted to be an artist, which made him feel different from the kids around him. Feeling different made him all the more anxious to please his peers and get their approval. He was a bright kid and it didn't take long for him to figure out how to keep the kids liking him. He watched to see what the "cool" ones did, and then he imitated it, as most kids who feel insecure about themselves do.

Fortunately, Kay knew who Joe was. She had spent hours in his classroom helping out with various activities in elementary school. She had seen him interact with friends. She knew his weaknesses and his strengths. She had learned from watching him at an early age where he was vulnerable. Now, rather than backing out of his life, as many parents are prone to do during the teen years, she became determined to move closer in. She instinctively knew that staying connected to him during these very toughest of years was more important than ever before, because his personality would make him more vulnerable than other kids to unhealthy temptations.

During one period, he wanted to dabble with smoking dope. When he started to date, he struggled with his desire to become sexually active. How did she know he was struggling with these things? She kept talking with him, asking questions; she kept a close eye on him; and she created activities they could do together—even when he resisted.

When it came to sex, she was particularly keen and watchful. And she became strict in her home. She communicated to Joe that she really liked his girlfriend, but that sex was risky stuff. She told him that he needed to wait and talked to him about the benefits of waiting until he was older. Then, she clearly told him that he wasn't to be home alone with his girlfriend because that might simply prove too tempting for him and she didn't want him to have to struggle with that. While many parents might expect Joe to sneak behind his mother's back, he never did. He told me that he thought his mother was right. Staying away from sex was hard for him and she had a point.

What worked was not the boundaries she set, but how she set them. He knew that she loved him, and she was very straightforward, honest, and firm. She also spoke to Joe as though she fully expected that he could abide by the rules. This made him feel good, he said.

Not everything ran smoothly, of course. Relationships rarely do. I'll never forget Joe sitting in my office one day complaining about his mother. "She just drives me absolutely crazy sometimes. She makes me angry, and we fight. But I know she really loves me," he said. In fact, when people have real love for each other, arguing can become another way to deepen their connection.

Joe is 19 now, and still a virgin. He credits his mom. Kay decided to stay emotionally connected to Joe and it worked.

DEVELOPING GREAT RELATIONSHIPS WITH OUR TEENS

If you want to develop connectedness with your teen, start by getting to know the world he lives in. Where he goes at night and who comes home with him after school. Who his friends are, what they do when they're together, what he likes, dislikes, his dreams, wishes, and wants.

It's a tough line to walk because he may think you're being suspicious of him rather than simply interested, but it's a line we must walk. You can take solace in the fact that you're not alone. Many of us have become confused about what to do, what to say, and when to say it when we're talking with our teens. Perhaps we have backed off from our teens' lives because we've heard too many "experts," like Benjamin Spock and T. Berry Brazelton, talk about the dangers of failing to meet the needs of young kids. By the time they reach adolescence, we're afraid to set limits, challenge them, or do anything else that might upset them. Maybe we're afraid that if we push them too far, they'll tell us they don't really want or need us. Or maybe they seem so emotionally complex and challenging that we just don't feel competent to deal with them. Whatever our fears, we need to understand that our kids need us, and we must have the courage to re-enter their world and their lives.

Fortunately, we don't have to feel completely lost on the journey. There is a road map. It leads us through four major landmarks: communication, intimacy, love, and appreciation.

CONNECTING THROUGH COMMUNICATION

It's no secret that teens want to communicate. They talk on the phone endlessly, instant-message each other for hours, and spend entire days hanging out with peers. The trick is getting them to communicate with you. It's easier than you might think. Take the fundamental steps listed below, and you'll be surprised at how quickly your teen will open up to you.

Like Your Teenager

If teenagers think you like them, they will communicate with you. If they think you dislike them, they will shut you out. It is imperative that you let your teen know that you like the person she is. This doesn't mean you have to agree with everything she does or says. Teens can deal with your disapproval, so long as they know that you accept and love them despite their flaws.

Understandably, liking your teen can be very difficult if you constantly argue with her, and you may feel estranged if your child is constantly away from home or online communicating with friends. Some parents just give up, and it's hard to blame them. Teenagers can be bitter, walled off, and hostile. I know because I've worked with numerous kids who are like that. As the physician for a halfway house for girls, I've spent hundreds of hours talking with kids who have been raped, beaten, abandoned, and emotionally starved. They arrive in my office hissing like cornered alley cats, and believe me, it's not easy to look past the cursing and obnoxiousness to the hurting, depressed girl underneath.

The key to liking unlikable teens lies in refusing to rise to the bait of their challenges. You have to remain calm and objective enough not to take their comments or attitudes personally. First of all, remember that you are not responsible for their obnoxious behaviors. When our children behave in ways we don't like, we often blame ourselves and feel responsible for changing that behavior on the spot. Don't. Let it go. It's not your fault. Kids are who they are and you need to accept that—for your own sake as well as theirs.

It may help to simply remind yourself that obnoxiousness is a symptom of something that's bothering your teen. If your child showed symptoms of diabetes, you would certainly be able to deal with him in a loving way. You can do the same in this situation.

You might also try picking out one or two qualities you admire in your teenager and then telling her what they are. If you're uncomfortable saying these things face to face, write a note and put it on her desk or pillow. She may throw the note away, call you a liar, or simply refuse to acknowledge your effort. That's okay. Wait a week and do it again. Don't fight back. Be determined to communicate that you genuinely like her. If you have a particularly volatile or distant relationship with your teen, this could take a year, but you can't give up. Your adolescent has a primal need to be liked and loved, and if you don't break through, someone else will. Chances are, that person won't be as nice as you.

Remember, time is on your side. Be determined to stay emotionally connected with your teen and don't back off even though everything inside you wants to give him the emotional (and physical) boot. When he realizes that nothing he can do or say will shake you loose, he'll begin to back off. After a while, he'll circle back around to you and see the emotional cord tied between the two of you. He may try desperately to break it for a while, but if you refuse to let it break, he will come back to you. You may have to wait until he's older to see this happen, but if you're patient, it will.

Listen to Your Teenager

Once your adolescent is willing to stay in the room with you for longer than 15 seconds (because he knows you really want to be with him), the most important principle in communication is to listen. Listening is important for two reasons: It gets you out of your own world and into his so you can learn what he sees, feels, thinks, and worries about. And if you're a good listener, over time your teenager will begin to listen to *you* because he feels important to you and liked by you.

So stop talking. Listen. Even if you don't like what you hear, listen. Somewhere in the words and sentences are reflections of what's happening in your child's heart. Is she bitter and angry all the time? Then she hurts. Does he continually talk about one or two people? Then there is a relationship you need to know about.

If your objective as you communicate is to teach them a lesson, give them "a piece of your mind," or straighten them out, you will lose them. The only way to accomplish those things is to listen. Then listen again and again.

Here's an experiment to try. For one week, every time you inter-act with your teen in conversation, keep your mouth closed and look him in the face when he talks. Rather than give your opinion, respond by asking why he feels the way he feels. You can ask any other nonjudgmental question that occurs to you—anything that comes out of genuine curiosity—but otherwise, be quiet. Your teen will be so thrown off, so excited that he is being heard, that he will return again and again for more conversation.

There are numerous ways to improve your listening skills.

Time your conversations well. Find a space in her world into which you can step. In the evening when your daughter is alone, approach her and ask simple questions about her life. Meet her for lunch away from school. Stay up an extra half-hour at night to talk with her.

Make eye contact. As she talks, look her in the eyes. Close the magazine, turn off the television, stop cooking. Eye contact is very intimate and hard to ignore. When you make eye contact, you connect.

Don't interrupt. I live in a family of talkers. This is good for me because I love to listen. People reveal everything about their desires, quirkiness, secret wishes, and vulnerabilities when given an opportunity to be heard. But the members of my family like to talk so much that they constantly interrupt one another. This drives me crazy, because as a listener, I want to hear the end of a person's sentence. When you interrupt your teenager, you're saying: "I don't want to hear the rest of what you're saying because either it's not important enough, or what I have to say is more important." Remember, teens are more emotionally sensitive and labile than we. No matter how badly you want to interrupt and correct, wait. It will pay off.

Sit down. Sitting while you talk communicates that what your teenager is saying is important to you, that you really want to hear it. So when the two of you begin a conversation, pull up a chair. If you're standing in the kitchen, sit up on the counter. If your child is sitting on the floor, don't be shy about joining him there.

Ask personal questions. Teens are egocentric and think about themselves constantly. So the best way to begin communicating is to ask them questions about themselves. Ask what they were doing after school, not because you're suspicious, but because you want to know them better. Find out what movies they've been watching lately. Ask who they like to be with and why. If you persistently, gently, and sincerely ask questions, your child will respond and open up. It might not happen in two days or even two weeks, but it probably will within a couple of months.

CONNECTING THROUGH INTIMACY

Communication opens the door for relationships. Intimacy cements them together. A psychologist friend of mine once explained intimacy in this way: "Intimacy means 'INTO-ME-SEE.' " How simple and true. Essentially, there are three types of intimacy—physical, emotional, and spiritual. We will examine the first two.

The Magic Touch

Some parents roll their eyes when they learn that teens need physical intimacy. Personal experience has taught them the opposite. A father retreats the first time his 13-year-old daughter shudders and stiffens when he gives her his usual hug. The body language of most teens toward parents seems to say, "Get away, your touch is creepy." Some parents liken hugging their teen to hugging a tree or a telephone pole. My own teenage son aims the top of his head toward my face when I ask for a goodnight kiss. Discomfort with their own bodies and with their sexuality makes them feel naturally awkward around their parents.

But teens still need physical intimacy as badly as ever. Just stand outside your local high school when the bell rings and watch the kids pour out. They hang all over each other. Boys paw at girls (no, it's not all sexual) and girls braid one another's hair or hug each other. My 18-year-old attends a youth group, where they are constantly hugging. Sometimes 20 or so kids will form a circle, hold hands, and yell "group hug!" Then all 20 run to the center of the circle for a giant hug. It's not sexual satisfaction they're looking for through this touching, but intimacy.

Touch lets teenagers know that someone sees them, someone likes them. So when a parent—still the most important person in a teen's life—touches them, it affects them deeply. Through physical contact, teenagers also learn self-respect, appropriate touch, body boundaries, and modesty.

If the teen in your home really is averse to hugging, start with safer touch. Touch her shoulder or her hair. Do it quickly, gently, and repeatedly. Be respectful and understand that some kids need to learn how to accept touch. Needless to say, never allow anyone to touch your child in a sexual way. This will confuse them deeply, cause them to reject healthy physical intimacy, and profoundly confuse their sexuality. If you find out that an adult friend or family member has touched your teen in a sexual way or even talked to him or her in a sexually provocative manner, deal with it immediately.

One other note: If you're a mother, it may feel more natural to hug your daughter, but it's equally important that you reach out to your son. Teen boys have a special need for a mother's love, and healthy touch keeps them connected to that love. If you're a father, it's just as important that you keep hugging your daughter. She needs to learn that she is to be handled gently and respectfully if she is to develop a healthy sexuality.

Creating Emotional Intimacy

Emotional intimacy occurs when a teenager feels a parent has "seen into" her true self and accepted what is there. If your teenager anticipates that she's going to meet with disapproval or rejection by mom or dad, she will hide that part. For example, if a girl is upset about excess weight gain but has heard her mother make critical remarks about overweight girls, she's unlikely to bring the subject up for discussion. But when she hides a portion of herself in that way, intimacy cannot occur.

The key to establishing emotional intimacy with your kids is creating an environment where they feel safe about expressing their feelings. Parents who yell a lot, who constantly criticize, who are unpredictable, or who get drunk will have difficulty establishing this emotional intimacy, particularly if they make their kids feel stupid or defensive. Teens with these types of parents naturally assume that exposing deeply personal thoughts and feelings is like asking to get trampled.

So how do you create a safe space? By spending more time with your kids, for one thing. Teens need our presence. When we give our kids time, it powerfully communicates that we love them. When friends, work, or anything else takes too much time away from our kids, they feel less loved. Try to be there for them when they leave for school and come home in the afternoons. Be there for meals and bedtime. Set aside a couple of hours every week that you can devote totally to them, with no interruptions. Think of activities you can share, like playing a sport or going to a movie. And the benefits of spending time won't fall only to your teen. You may find that your own child will turn out to be one of the best companions you could imagine.

In addition to time, you must provide a safe location for emotional intimacy, a place where your child feels comfortable expressing his thoughts and feelings without interruptions or eavesdropping. Maybe it's his bedroom, or the family den, or the back porch. So long as your teen feels at ease, protected, and secure, anyplace will do.

I met a gentleman recently who told me how he connects with his kids. Every year, he rents a house in Europe for one month, and he, his wife, and their two teenagers spend the time together. No friends. No television. No work. Just one another. What did they do while they were there? I asked.

At first, of course, everyone cried that they were bored and wanted to go home, but that was out of the question. They had to work together to figure out what to do. That's how connectedness developed. They looked at empty time and space together and figured out how to fill it. They were edgy and irritable for awhile because they didn't know how to work together. They didn't know how to negotiate, communicate, or compromise. But they learned through struggling.

They came to enjoy hiking together, shopping together, and even cooking together. They read, put together puzzles, and organized day trips for sightseeing. They learned each other's likes and dislikes because each person got to choose and organize different activities. The point is, when they removed all of the "stuff" that separated them (sports, work, TV, etc.) they naturally developed connectedness.

CONNECTING THROUGH LOVE

When we think of Mother Teresa, we inevitably think about her boundless ability to love others and to act on that love. There was nothing complicated about it. As she walked the filthy streets of Calcutta, she looked for people in need. When she found them, she touched them in the most intimate places on their bodies—their faces. We could see her press her frail palms against their cheeks, capturing their gaze and offering hers in return. She made love simple, identifying and then filling the needs of those she saw *without expecting anything in return.*

This is the kind of unconditional love you need to give your teenagers. You must love your child whether or not he or she returns the favor. It is the greatest gift you can give, and it will yield great blessings to both you and your child. If a teen makes herself difficult to love, so much the better. In the end, she will benefit that much more from your love.

I remember one extremely sick girl with anorexia nervosa. She made it harder for me to love her than any other teenager I'd ever treated. Whenever I opened my mouth or approached her, she snarled venomously and swore at me. When I firmly but gently told her swearing at me was not acceptable, she simply hissed. She was so walled off that even simple expressions of kindness were hard to give. Sometimes I just wanted to stand up, tell her we were done, that she was hopeless and mean, and that she had to find herself a new doctor. But being loving toward her meant seeing beneath the hissing and the icy glares to the tiny, crying little girl inside who was stuck in an iron cage of self-hatred. I knew she couldn't escape unless someone loved her. That didn't mean I let her walk all over me, of course. And it didn't mean I needed to tolerate her self-destructive behavior. In fact, I set firm boundaries. She was not to curse at me. If she couldn't stop, she would have to find another doctor. If she refused to eat or insisted on exercising every day, she would be sent to a hospital. No ifs, ands, or buts. I knew that she could use her eating problems to manipulate the people around her, and I wasn't about to give in to that. I gave her strict rules, but I also expressed my love for her. Eventually, she left her anorexia behind and turned into one of the sweetest people you could ever meet.

Just as I learned to love that young woman, parents must look beneath the obnoxious, childish, selfish, and confused behavior our teenagers often express and continue to provide our love through patience and kind words. This, of course, means we also have to give up our own obnoxious, childish, selfish, and confused behavior, which is not an easy task for many of us. However, we have to do our best. If we can't offer our love in an adult way but rather give love only to get something in return, kids will intuitively sense this and pull away. I often see this situation among the children of divorced parents.

One of my patients, Shelby, was a 15-year-old girl whose father had left her mother for another woman. Shortly afterward, Shelby began spending weekends with him. He bought her clothes and a car (before she could drive), but insisted that she spend time with him and his new girlfriend. Obviously, he wanted something from his daughter. She told me she hated her time with her father and deeply resented his pressuring her to spend time with his girlfriend. She knew the only reason he gave her attention and gifts was so that she would approve of his behavior, but she felt that what her dad was doing was wrong.

Shelby knew that his love was conditional, and in her mind, invalid. She needed her dad—his time, his genuine love. He didn't want to give it because, quite simply, he wanted his girlfriend more. Now, three years later, Shelby rarely sees her dad and lives with a large vacancy in her heart. To no one's surprise, she has had a string of boyfriends and sexual relationships.

Love is tough. It means sacrificing for our kids and loving them not because of what we can get from them—approval, fulfillment of dreams, feeling better about our parenting, whatever—but because those are the very things they need from us.

CONNECTING THROUGH APPRECIATION

Appreciation is a word we use to describe our recognition of someone else's value or worth. We all need to feel valuable to the people we know and the world we live in, but teens, who naturally struggle with insecurities about their developing identities, feel this need even more keenly than other people do. Finding this sense—that they have traits and talents other people appreciate—makes them feel good, acceptable, loved, and defined. Parents, especially, should do everything they can to help their adolescents feel valuable and valued. Otherwise, teens will turn to peers, media, or relationships outside the family for a sense of what makes them valuable, and as we've already seen, the answer they're likely to get can be summed up in one word: sex.

So think about it: What will you tell your child to make him or her feel valued? If the answer seems elusive, then rephrase it this way: What are the traits I really love about my child? You must be able to answer this question more for your kids than for yourself.

Before you answer, however, let me offer one caveat: When I say "traits," I don't mean academic, sports, or artistic accomplishments.

At issue *isn't what they've done; it's who they are.* We've all seen sports parents who show up at every game cheering their child's victories but completely losing their composure—and sometimes their temper—over their child's failures. When teenagers see our enthusiasm swell *only* when they excel at something, they think their performance increases our love for them. Then—and this hurts—they become stuck performing, studying, or producing to earn more expressions of love from us. Is this what we want for our children? Or do we want them to know that they are fundamentally, at the very core of who they are, lovable and valuable to us?

If you praise your son's great soccer abilities, also praise his patience. If your daughter is as compassionate or perceptive as she is bright, give her as much credit for the former qualities as for the latter. Recognize courage, persistence, wisdom, gratefulness, self-control, compassion, kindness, faithfulness, joy, and goodness in your children. They deserve it.

PARENTAL DISAPPROVAL OF SEX

There are four main reasons teenagers have sex, and none of them are healthy or lead to good relationships:

For fun, excitement, and thrills; to seek out the unknown. In this situation, most teens have very limited attachments to their sexual partners, viewing him or her as an object of play. Teens who engage in sex strictly as a game become increasingly detached and emotionally distant from their partners.

To be accepted by peers and society at large. We know that young teens typically have poor self-esteem, and that some teens opt for sex to bolster their sense of value. Kids who are immersed in media are particularly vulnerable to engaging in sex to feel accepted.

To have their needs met. All teens are wired with needs for intimacy, love, and a sense of their own value. When these needs are not met in meaningful ways through relationships with family and loved ones, a teen may turn to sex to fill those voids.

To lose themselves. Some teens use sex like a drug to blot out pain or other uncomfortable feelings. When having sex doesn't work and the pain continues or gets worse, the only way these kids know how to cope is by trying again, only harder, more frequently, and with different partners.

In my experience, the latter two reasons account for most early sexual activity among teenagers. Basically, teens are having sex to find something missing in their lives. They're desperate for a connection with the adults around them, primarily their parents.

As parents, most of us know these things instinctively. Some of us may feel shy or uncomfortable communicating our disapproval of teen sex to our kids. Still, we feel it deep down, and communicate it we must because, as the Add Health study shows, a significant factor in keeping teenagers from becoming sexually active is perceived parental disapproval. If a son knows that his parents don't think he should have sex, he is more likely to wait than if they give him a pocketful of condoms.

Parents' convictions and beliefs change the behavior of their kids. Why? Because teenagers want to love and be loved by their parents. They want to please them in order to get that love—to stay "hooked" to them. They figure out what their parents want and believe and respond to it. This deep dynamic drives their behavior much more than anything they learn in a sex ed classroom.

So parents (and other significant adults) must define their own convictions about teenagers and sex. If you're not sure, ask your teen. She may not be able to tell you your favorite color or food, but she knows how you feel about almost everything else. She knows what you believe about her and sex, dating, and birth control. And she knows that if you believe it's okay for her to be sexually active (even if you haven't articulated that message to her yourself), then she has the green light to be sexually active.

For parents who care for their children and want to protect them, there is perhaps no better or stronger force at their disposal than connectedness. And remember, the connection takes place on both sides of the relationship. While your teens will benefit profoundly through feeling a deep sense of connection with you, you may be surprised at the sense of love, satisfaction, and vitality you will feel through your connection with them.

TWELVE

■ If you have sex with six people by the time you're 20 years old, and they have had the same number of partners as you, you've been exposed to the diseases of 63 people. If you have sex with seven people, you've been exposed to the diseases of 127 people.

Holding Off

DESPITE ALL THE BAD NEWS, I STILL have hope. Why? Because teens are great. They're smart, they're passionate, they know how to laugh, and, when given half a chance, they make good judgments. It's the culture they're immersed in that brings them down, a culture that makes money by using sex to sell them movies, clothing, CDs, and even candy bars. Our teens are literally being trained into sexual activity, indoctrinated into a lifestyle that can kill them. Fortunately, the culture doesn't have the last word. *We do.* Parents, teachers, grandparents, and everyone else who cares for, worries about, and loves teens.

If the data seems discouraging, take a second look. It's true that studies have found about 40% of high school freshmen are sexually active. But that means 60%, over half, have decided to wait. In fact, nearly the same number of tenth-graders, about half of eleventh-graders, and four in ten high school seniors remain virgins. That's great news, not just because the kids who are waiting aren't exposed to disease, but because it tells us that *any* teen can make healthy choices if he or she wants to. We need to look at these kids who aren't having sex and ask what they are doing that helps them see through the media blitz and stay true to themselves.

As it turns out, they're holding off for a variety of reasons. First, some teens are smart enough to be afraid of pregnancy or getting an STD. This fear can be very healthy, but we must be careful that it doesn't lead our teens into believing that sex is bad or grotesque when they learn about its accompanying dangers.

I saw this happen to Tamara. When she was in the eighth grade, she learned in her sex education class about the mechanics of sex, STDs, and condoms. She even had to practice putting condoms on bananas. She said that she felt so "grossed out" by it all that she didn't want anything to do with boys.

While these feelings are normal for many 13-year-olds, Tamara's stayed with her well into her later teen years. She refused to date during high school or college. Even her friendships with boys were strained, she later told me. Unfortunately, Tamara didn't divulge her feeling to anyone about sex until she was older (college-age). With some help talking things through with a close adult, she was able to see sex in a more positive light.

So we need to strike a healthy balance with kids. They should feel fearful about having sex at an early age because of pregnancy and STDs, but we should also teach them that it's something very special, beautiful, and worth waiting for.

Not all teens postpone sexual activity out of fear. Some do because they simply don't want the complications it brings into their lives. Many have told me that it makes relationships more serious, more committed, and they don't feel ready to deal with those issues. This, in my judgment, is mature and sound reasoning and I encourage teens who tell me this to keep going.

I have to say, I am always impressed with kids like Todd. He is 18 and has had a few girlfriends but has never been sexually active with any of them. He loves the outdoors and is intense about basketball. He says that ever since he was little, he wanted to be a professional basketball player. At first he didn't want to become sexually involved with his girlfriends because he took his athletics seriously and was afraid that spending more time (which would naturally follow sex because the intensity of the relationship would increase) with his girlfriends would give him less time for his sports. Then, when he got older, he felt good about not having sex for other reasons. He saw his friends involved in "one-night stands" as well as being sexually active with more serious girlfriends. Either way, he said, he saw that they struggled with worry about pregnancy, and he was turned off by the way their attitudes toward girls and themselves changed. In short, Todd liked being different. He liked the fact that his life felt uncomplicated and this worked well for him. Kids like Todd are all around us. All they need is encouragement and some strong, healthy messages from us.

There is another group of teens who are holding off having sex. These are the kids who do so because they have high regard for it. They believe that it is not a social event; it is private and special. They have developed a tremendous respect for their own bodies and feelings, neither of which they're willing to share at random. Rather than feel embarrassed about being different from many of their peers, they seem to like who they are.

Sometimes I ask kids how they have come to feel this way. Almost universally, they tell me that their parents have taught them to respect themselves. What is particularly interesting to me is that they may not fully comprehend what that means or what the long-term implications are, but they believe what their parents teach them, they like it, and they put it into action. This is much like teaching our kids to say "thank you" when they're little. We teach them because we want them to feel and show appreciation. Usually, the ability to actually feel appreciation follows much later developmentally, but we train them anyway, knowing that their rote behavior may eventually translate into real gratitude. This is very much the way teens come to really respect themselves. When they are taught the simple mechanics at first, eventually they come to feel it and live it on a much more meaningful level.

It's really not so hard for parents to communicate self-respect to teens. They want positive messages—about themselves, about life, and about sex. They don't want to feel used, manipulated by a girl-friend or boyfriend. They want someone to tell them that their bodies are beautiful, so beautiful in fact that they should keep them protected and covered. This is not a shame issue, it is quite the opposite. Teens who like their bodies care for them and expose them only to special people at certain times. They naturally understand the issue. After all, they keep their cars tuned up, waxed, in the garage, parked carefully, and locked. If they can have that kind of respect for their cars, they can certainly have it for themselves.

There are only two reasons that parents or teachers would not aggressively teach teens to postpone sex until they are well beyond their teen or young adult years: either they believe that teens *don't really need* to wait or they believe that teens *are unable* to wait.

Neither is true.

First, sexual activity must be delayed. Teens who have sex are playing with fire. As we've seen, their bodies aren't physiologically ready, their minds aren't cognitively or physiologically ready, and condoms, at best, only partially reduce the risk of some, not all, STDs.

Second, teenagers are perfectly capable of controlling their own behavior. In fact, with issues like smoking cigarettes, we absolutely expect it of them. We don't hand out filtered cigarettes to kids, assuming they will eventually smoke because they can't help themselves, and therefore our job is to help decrease their risk of getting lung cancer by filtering out a few, not all, of the toxins. We tell kids, "Don't smoke, because it will kill you." We should be telling them the same thing about having sex while they're still teenagers.

TEACHING KIDS TO POSTPONE SEX

As we've seen, parents can significantly influence a teen's behavior far more than peers can. Teens and parents have stronger emotional bonds. When kids argue with their parents, they feel deeper pain than they do over conflicts with peers, and joy shared with a parent goes deeper than happiness shared with a friend. You rarely hear about people going to a psychological therapist because of some trauma caused by friends. They go to heal emotional scars they believe were caused by parents. Bottom line: Parents have extraordinary power in their kids' lives.

Nowhere is this power more influential than when it comes to making sexual decisions. A national survey taken by The National Campaign to Prevent Teen Pregnancy[1] asked teens the following question: "When it comes to your sexual decision making, which is most influential: the media, friends, teachers and sex educators, brothers and sisters, religious organizations or parents?" Surprise! *Thirty-eight percent* said that their parents influenced them most. Friends influenced 31%, religious organizations influenced 9%, siblings 7%, teachers 6%, and the media 3%.

The problem is, most parents hate talking about sexual issues with their kids. They are embarrassed, insecure, and often just don't know what to say. But what happens when parents fail to say anything? Teens feel that parents don't care one way or the other. Many kids will just go ahead and become sexually active.

There is no need to be timid. You can influence your children's attitude about sex without diving into gritty details. What's really important *isn't what you say*, but *what you believe*. Children (particularly younger ones) are anxious to please their parents because they want to feel loved and accepted by you. They figure out very quickly what you like, dislike, approve of, and disapprove of.

Take dieting, for example. If a teen girl hears her mother comment on other women's beautiful *and thin* figures repeatedly, she quickly realizes that being thin is important to her mother. Because she wants her mother's approval, she'll try to maintain a thin physique. If she is chubby, however, she will feel disapproval from her mother and her self-esteem will suffer. She will feel these feelings even if her mother never says a word about her personally.

With sexual activity, the same principle holds. From the time our children are young, we must give them lessons that their bodies are precious and not to be shared too soon or indiscriminately with other people. Beginning around age four, when I examine the genitalia of a young patient, I tell him or her to remember that "private areas" are very special and that only a doctor, mom, or dad should be able to see them. Then, I make sure to drape their groin with a paper cloth to enforce the notion of privacy. I am a stickler about covering children's private areas in hospitals or in exam rooms rather than expose them—even to the eyes of their siblings. Small gestures like this communicate to kids that privacy and personal boundaries are good things.

As children grow older and you watch movies or television programs with them, comment on how characters they see do and do not respect their bodies. During scenes where unmarried people are having sex, ask your kids how much they believe those people value their bodies, their sexuality. Then let them know that you want better for your children, that their sexuality, their bodies, are too important to be shared randomly, even with people they think they love. As they move into the teen years, periodically reiterate that you like their strong body, that you want them to regard it as special and private, and that you believe they are strong enough to make their own healthy decisions and not to follow the crowd. Your positive attitude will make your child feel good about herself, whether she shows it or not, and high self-esteem begets enlightened self-interest, which allows kids to set firm boundaries according to their beliefs.

If you are at all able to dive into the details, sometime around age 11, one or both parents should openly discuss sexual issues in a respectful and honest manner with their child. Just remain sensitive to your teen's discomfort with the topic. Talking about sex with kids can be embarrassing for both parents and kids, but believe me, your child may be far more uncomfortable than you are. Keep your conversations simple and direct. If you aren't sure about the answer to a question your child poses, don't fake it. Tell him that his question was a good one and you'll find the answer for him. Also, be sure to talk to him in private. Nobody wants a brother or sister hanging around when talking to a parent about sex.

Be sensitive to your child's maturity level. Some kids will be ready to talk about being sexually active versus postponing sex when they are 10, others won't be ready until they are 14. Talk about birth control so your kids will understand the risks involved with using it. Tell them that condoms aren't the answer and give them statistics to back up your points. Tell them about STDs, but be positive. Try to make sex look not like a bad thing, but like a wonderful pleasure that must be greatly respected.

When your child is younger and starting to ask questions about sex, give him simple, straightforward answers. As he grows older and begins to learn about sex at school, tell him that you want to help him understand everything that he is hearing and that you want to be his final information source. What he's hearing is so important that you want to be sure he understands it. When he learns about STDs, ask him what he's learned, just as you would ask what book he's reading in English. Be matter-of-fact. If he's learning about chlamydia and herpes, let him know that they are real and that they shouldn't be a part of his life. One of the best things you can do is get hold of his sex education curriculum. Most teachers are happy to have interested parents. Look it over. If films are shown, don't go in and watch them in class with your teen, but ask to see them on your own sometime. The most important thing is to stay abreast of what your teen or young child is hearing at school so that you can reinforce the positives and let him know that sex is serious business.

Don't hide anything. Just because you don't believe your child should be using condoms, for example, doesn't mean you should skirt the subject. Just let her know that condoms, if used perfectly every time, will prevent pregnancy but not STDs, and that many other problems can come from sexual activity at her age. I have found that teens who get that kind of information are less likely to use birth control early on.

AMBIVALENCE IS PERMISSION

If after all this you don't believe your teenagers should stay away from sex, or if you act ambivalently toward their having sex, they won't stay away from it. And if a parent doesn't believe teenagers can control their sexual drives, they won't. I've seen teens who receive positive reinforcement about refraining from sex from their parents take the message and run with it. But I have also seen teens who receive ambivalent messages.

Here is what, in my experience, typically happens with many parents of my generation. Let's say a girl, Susan, brings home a boyfriend when she's 16. Her boyfriend, Tom, is 18, cute, and very polite. He doesn't swear, his grades are pretty good, and he seems like a safe driver. Mom and Dad like him. They trust him to be careful with Susan. They wonder to themselves whether or not the two are sexually active but don't worry too much because they can't imagine that Tom would give Susan an STD (he sure doesn't look like he'd be the kind of kid to sleep around, they think). Besides, both kids have had sex education at school, so they'll be responsible and "safe." In other words, they trust the kids to wear condoms if they do have sex.

Now let me tell you what Susan says to me when the doors are closed. She tells me that she and Tom started having sex three weeks after they started dating and she believes that her parents don't suspect anything. She believes that if she told her parents, one wouldn't care (usually the mother) and would want her on birth control. The other parent might get mad, but would ultimately feel relieved that she was being "responsible" by using condoms. When I ask what her parents really think about her having sex, she's not sure. Susan tells me that they've never really had a heart-to-heart conversation about it, but she does know that her parents had sex before they were married. (This is fairly common. Parents frequently divulge their sexual pasts with their teens. Be careful. While you don't want to hide anything, your business is private and it just might encourage your teen to make mistakes that could cost her dearly.)

In short, Susan tells me that she started having sex with Tom because she just didn't think it was "that big of a deal" and her parents never made much of it.

There are way too many Susans sleeping with nice guys like Tom who are only doing so because no one, *no one*, has told them why and how they should postpone sexual relationships until they're older.

Ambivalent messages come from parents three ways:

Silence. When we say nothing about the importance of waiting, our kids, like Susan, feel that they might as well try it. This is the most common form of ambivalence I see, and I believe that it stems from a genuine lack of understanding on the parent's part of the serious consequences of sex that our teens face. We believe that the dangers for our kids aren't much different from the ones we faced 20 or 30 years ago. Parents simply let teens make decisions about sexual activity because they believe that nothing terribly bad will happen.

Poor example. Time and time again teens tell me that their single mother or father warns them that they shouldn't be sexually active, but that same mother or father is living, unmarried, with a sexual partner—often one of a long line of partners. What teens in this situation ask me is that since their mother or father is clearly sexually active, why shouldn't they be? In fact, the kids have an excellent point. If a parent really wants his or her teen to stay away from sex, there are some serious decisions to make. If a parent stops having sex in order to provide a good example for their teen, believe me, that teen will sit up and take notice!

Inconsistency. Parents who warn their child that teen sex isn't good but spend a lot of time watching highly sexualized television or movies are muddying the waters. While this may not seem like an ambivalent message to us, it can be for teens. If a kid sees his parent "approving" of sex between young sophisticated singles on television, why shouldn't he be one of those young sophisticated singles?

My personal experience with teens has led me to know that many of these "double messages" lead teens toward sexual activity.

Fortunately, while many parents remain ambivalent about teenage sex, many teens are not. It's time we began encouraging and applauding the wisdom of teens who show mature good judgment about living sexually healthy lives. We need to realize that not only *should* teens wait to have sex, but that many *want* to wait and need to be told *how* to wait.

We can start by setting clear, unambivalent standards for our children, in what we say and what we do. If that makes you cringe, get over it. Parents worry that by communicating clearly that sex should be saved for adulthood, they will alienate their kids. But just the *opposite* will happen. Kids like having someone they love set high standards because it demonstrates faith that they can meet those standards. We are not shy about setting the bar high in other areas, such as education and taking drugs. We need the same attitude where sex is concerned.

IT'S NEVER TOO LATE

I often see teens in my office who have had sex with one or many partners and want to stop. They've learned hard lessons from contracting an STD or suffering depression, but they feel that they are already "damaged goods." They feel that they have lost their virginity, or the healthy body or healthy emotional state they had before and don't feel that they can recover either of these things. If they want their old body back, I treat whatever disease they have and if it's gone, I tell them that they can start all over again. If they have herpes, I help them learn to deal with it and teach them that they too can become "secondary virgins."

This may sound ridiculous to the adult mind, but I have found it to be extremely important for some teens. They want to leave their mistakes behind, so I try to help them do this. I try to teach them to leave sex behind and start fresh. I encourage them as truthfully as I can that they are physically healthy (if they are), then encourage them to deal head-on with the emotional fallout they have encountered from being sexually active and move forward. Teens want and need second chances to start on a new path to sexual health, and I feel that I, as their advocate, must help them do this. There is no reason parents can't do the same for them.

Not all sexually active kids come to me wanting to stop having sex, of course, but just as I would try to get any smoker to quit smoking, I feel it's my responsibility to try to get kids to give up their unhealthy lifestyle choices as well. My methods don't always prove popular, but I've given them a lot of thought.

There are basically three groups of teens. Those who won't become sexually active, those who are considering becoming sexually active but who will listen to me or another adult, and those who are determined to become sexually active and won't listen to any advice to the contrary.

I educate the first group about the risks of STDs and depression, applaud their decision to hold off, and help them devise a plan to do so.

I question members of the second group about their thoughts on sex and teach them about the risks. I'm tougher on this group, "reading them the riot act" and hammering home the message that they're playing with fire. If they're already sexually active and are willing to work with me to stop having sex, but aren't quite ready to give it up, I make them a deal. I tell them that as their physician who cares about them, I can't let them continue such a dangerous activity. I tell them my goal is to get them to stop having sex within the next six months. During that time, I see them in my office every two weeks for a brief visit to help them accomplish this goal. In the meantime, they must be "as safe as possible" and use condoms. I also tell them that condoms are no answer. Interestingly, teens love this plan. Once they see that I take their behavior seriously, that I'm willing to see them repeatedly in my office, they begin taking their sexual behavior seriously and they comply! After six months, if a patient refuses to stop having sex, I tell them they need a new physician. Then I sign off.

The third group, kids who are determined to have sex no matter what, is the most challenging. I've found that most of these kids are struggling with depression. Their reasons for having sex go way beyond their sexual drives—generally their emotional needs are not being met. I try my best to get them to see a good therapist. I tell them about the serious risks they're taking and ask if they care that they're hurting themselves. Some tell me right to my face that they don't care and they won't stop. I tell them that if that's the deal, they either find a new doctor or agree to work with me for the six-month period. Again, most kids love this idea, particularly the attention I provide, and they agree to the six-month "weaning" period.

I keep them on birth control if they're already using it, and urge them to use condoms. (Unfortunately, most of the kids in this third group don't use condoms anyway, because they don't care about getting an STD. In fact, many of them have already had at least one.) I don't like doing this, but I really don't have any choice. Then, after six months, if they are still sexually active, I let them know that by being sexually active, they are going against my best medical advice.

I draw a clear line and offer to help them any way I can to change their behaviors. And I just try to be there for them.

Interestingly, most teens respond incredibly well. I've had very few patients leave my practice after the six months. My method tells them that their actions have immediate, serious consequences, and that someone in their life really cares about them.

These are the kids who are in deep psychological pain. They use their risky sexual behaviors to cope with this pain. I know that in one, two, or even three office visits, I can't take away their pain and I can't change their behavior. I have to accept my own limitations, and focus on the kids I *can* help.

IN CONCLUSION

Today's teens live during a time when sex can be toxic and life-threatening. They stand in the middle of an invisible battlefield surrounded by disease and depression, injury, and death. The only way to safety is to arm these children with knowledge so that they can make the right choices, and with strong character so those choices can be held firmly even in the face of the culture's sexual blitz.

Victories won't come from wearing condoms or swallowing birth control pills, but from wisdom, maturity, and self-control. These are lessons that only we, the adults in their lives, can teach them, through the very connections and relationships we forge with them.

Love your kids and have faith in them. There is no question that they will survive the battle. They will if we enter it with them and help them through the fight.

Notes

TWO

1. Joe S. McIlhaney, Jr., "Ignoring an Epidemic (Editorial)." Austin, Tex.: The Medical Institute for Sexual Health, *Media Advisories*. Internet on-line. www.medinstitute.org/media/editorial-1.htm.

2. Stuart Collins *et al.*, "High Incidence of Cervical Human Papillomavirus Infection in Women During Their First Sexual Relationship." *British Journal of Obstetrics and Gynecology* 109 (2002): 96-98.

3. National Center for HIV, STD, and TB Prevention, Centers for Disease Control, U.S. Department of Health and Human Services. "Tracking the Hidden Epidemics." Database on-line. www.cdc/gov.com.

4. ibid.

5. D. T. Fleming *et al.*, "Herpes Simplex Virus Type 2 in the United

States, 1976 to 1994." *New England Journal of Medicine* 337 (1997): 1105-1160.

6. See note 3 above.

7. See note 5 above.

8. ibid.

9. See note 3 above.

10. Thomas R. Eng and William T. Butler, eds., Committee on Prevention and Control of Sexually Transmitted Diseases, Institute of Medicine. *The Hidden Epidemic.* Washington, D.C.: National Academy Press, 1997.

11. J. Dennis Fortenberry, "Unveiling the Hidden Epidemic of Sexually Transmitted Diseases." *Journal of the American Medical Association* 287 (2002): 768-769.

12. See note 5 above.

13. ibid.

14. J. M. Walboomers *et al.*, "Human Papillomavirus Is a Necessary Cause of Invasive Cervical Cancer Worldwide." *Journal of Pathology* 189 (1999): 12-19.

15. J. Mork *et al.*, "Human Papillomavirus Infection as a Risk Factor for Squamous Cell Carcinoma of the Head and Neck." *New England Journal of Medicine* 15 (2001): 1125-1131.

16. "Young People At Risk: HIV/AIDS Among America's Youth." Center for Disease Control and Prevention. National Center for HIV, STD, and TB Prevention, Divisions of HIV/AIDS Prevention. Internet on-line. www.cdc.gov/hiv/pubs/facts/youth.htm.

17. ibid.

18. P. S. Rosenberg, R. J. Biggar, and J. J. Goedert, "Declining Age at HIV Infection in the United States" (letter). *New England Journal of Medicine* 330 (1994): 789-790.

19. A. E. Washington and P. Katz, "Cost and Payment Source for Pelvic Inflammatory Disease." *Journal of the American Medical Association* 266 (1991): 2565-2569.

20. See note 3 above.

21. "Know-It-All Teens." *Pediatrics for Parents* 18, no. 12 (2000): 9.

22. ibid.

23. *America's Youth: Measuring the Risk*, 4th ed. Washington, D.C.: The Institute for Youth Development, 2002.

24. C. Roberts and J. Pfister, "Increasing Proportion of HSV-1 as a Cause of Genital Herpes Infection in College Students." Presented at the 2002 National STD Prevention Conference, San Diego, Calif., March 4-7, 2002. Abstract no. LB1.

25. "Teens Say Oral Sex 'Doesn't Count' As More Engage." LifeDate, Spring 2001 issue. Internet on-line. www.lutheransforlife.org/lifedate/2001/spring/teens_say_oral_sex_doesnt_count.html.

26. Ja Rule. *Pain Is Love*. Compact disk recording. Murder Inc. Records, 2001.

27. Lil' Kim. *Notorious Kim*. Compact disk recording. Atlantic Records, 2000.

28. Kid Rock. *Devil Without a Cause*. Compact disk recording. Atlantic Records, 1998.

29. *Guidelines for Comprehensive Sexuality Education, Kindergarten-12th Grade*, 2nd ed. National Guidelines Task Force. New York: Sexuality Information and Education Council of the United States, 1996.

THREE

1. D. T. Fleming *et al.*, "Herpes Simplex Virus Type 2 in the United States, 1976 to 1994." *New England Journal of Medicine* 337 (1997): 1105-1160.

2. American Social Health Association. "Sexually Transmitted Disease in America: How Many Cases and at What Cost?" Menlo Park, Calif.: The Henry J. Kaiser Family Foundation, 1998.

   L. A. Koutsky and N. B. Kiviat, "Genital Human Papillomavirus" in: K. K. Holmes *et al.*, eds., *Sexually Transmitted Diseases*, 3rd ed. New York: McGraw-Hill, 1999, pp. 347-359.

3. "Human Papilloma Virus (HPV)—What Is It?" The Medical Institute for Sexual Health, Austin, Tex., *Sexual Health Update*. Spring 2000, vol. 8, no. 1.

4. National Center for HIV, STD, and TB Prevention, Centers for Disease Control, U.S. Department of Health and Human Services. "Tracking the Hidden Epidemics." Database on-line. www.cdc/gov.com.

5. ibid.

6. A. E. Washington and P. Katz, "Cost and Payment Source for Pelvic Inflammatory Disease." *Journal of the American Medical Association* 266 (1991): 2565-2569.

7. *"Sexual Health Today: Exploring the Past, Preserving the Future through Choices Today."* Slide Programs, Lecture Notes, and Supplemental Materials. Austin, Tex.: The Medical Institute for Sexual Health, 1998.

8. G. Paz-Bailey *et al.*, "Condom Protection Against STD: A Study Among Adolescents Attending a Primary Care Clinic in Atlanta." Presented at the 2002 National STD Prevention Conference, San Diego, Calif., March 4-7, 2002. Abstract B9D.

9. J. Abma, A. Chandra, W. Mosher, L. Peterson, and L. Piccinino, *Fertility, Family Planning and Women's Health: New Data from the 1995 National Survey of Family Growth*. National Center for Health Statistics, Centers for Disease Control and Prevention. Vital Health and Statistics Series no. 23 (19), 1997.

10. Harvey Elder, "HIV-2002." Presented at the Medical Institute for Sexual Health "Health on the Horizon" Conference. Palm Springs, Calif., June 2002. Available through www.medinstitute.org.

11. J. M. Walboomers *et al.*, "Human Papillomavirus Is a Necessary Cause of Invasive Cervical Cancer Worldwide." *Journal of Pathology* 189 (1999): 12-19.

12. Robert Greenlee, Taylor Murray, Sherry Bolden, and Phyllis A. Wingo, "Cancer Statistics, 2000." *CA: A Cancer Journal for Clinicians* 50 (2000): 7-33.

13. Robert D. Burk *et al.*, "Declining Prevalence of Cervicovaginal Human Papillomavirus Infection with Age is Independent of Other Risk Factors." *Sexually Transmitted Diseases* July-August, 1996.

14. See note 4 above.

15. L. A. Koutsky and N. B. Kiviat, "Genital Human Papillomavirus" in: K. K. Holmes *et al.*, eds., *Sexually Transmitted Diseases*, 3rd ed. New York: McGraw-Hill, 1999, pp. 347-359.

16. www.cdc.gov/std/hpv.

17. Stuart Collins *et al.*, "High Incidence of Cervical Human Papillomavirus Infection in Women During Their First Sexual Relationship." *British Journal of Obstetrics and Gynecology* 109 (2002): 96-98.

18. Thomas R. Eng and William T. Butler, eds., Committee on Prevention and Control of Sexually Transmitted Diseases, Institute of Medicine. *The Hidden Epidemic.* Washington, D.C.: National Academy Press, 1997.

19. J. Mork *et al.*, "Human Papillomavirus Infection as a Risk Factor for Squamous Cell Carcinoma of the Head and Neck." *New England Journal of Medicine* 15 (2001): 1125-1131.

20. www.adolescenthealth.org/cme/progam.hpv.

21. M. Schiftman and D. Solomon, "Findings to Date from the ASCUS-LSIL Triage Study (ALTS)," *Arch Path Lab Med*, 2003; 127: 946–49.

22. ibid.

23. R. L. Sweet and R. S. Gibbs, *Infectious Diseases of the Female Genital Tract*, 2nd ed. Baltimore: Williams & Wilkins, 1990, p. 145.

24. See note 1 above.

25. ibid.

26. G. J. Mertz, "Epidemiology of Genital Herpes Infections." *Infectious Diseases Clinics of North America* 7 (1993): 825-839.

27. Lawrence Corey and H. Hunter Handsfield, "Genital Herpes and Public Health." *Journal of the American Medical Association* 283 (2000): 791-794.

28. John Leo *et al.*, "The New Scarlet Letter: Herpes, An Incurable Virus, Threatens to Undo the Sexual Revolution." *Time*, 2 August 1982, 62-66.

29. D. N. Catotti, P. Clarke, and K. E. Catoe, "Herpes Revisited: Still a Cause of Concern." *Sexually Transmitted Diseases* 20 (1993): 77-80.

30. Centers for Disease Control and Prevention (1995, December). HIV/AIDS Surveillance Report 7(2), 5.

31. ibid.

32. See note 10 above.

33. See note 18 above.

34. Marilyn Billingsley, "Sexually Transmitted Liver Disease." Presented at the Medical Institute for Sexual Health "Health on the Horizon" Conference. Palm Springs, Calif., June 2002. Available through www.medinstitute.org.

35. ibid.

FOUR

1. National Center for HIV, STD, and TB Prevention, Centers for Disease Control, U.S. Department of Health and Human Services. "Tracking the Hidden Epidemics." Database on-line. www.cdc/gov.com.

2. ibid.

3. Thomas R. Eng and William T. Butler, eds., Committee on Prevention and Control of Sexually Transmitted Diseases, Institute of Medicine. *The Hidden Epidemic.* Washington, D.C.: National Academy Press, 1997.

4. Centers for Disease Control and Prevention (1996, September). Sexually Transmitted Disease Surveillance 1995, *Morbidity and Mortality Weekly Report* 7(2).

5. *"Sexual Health Today. Exploring the Past, Preserving the Future through Choices Today."* Slide Programs, Lecture Notes, and Supplemental Materials. Austin, Tex.: The Medical Institute for Sexual Health 1998.

6. See note 3 above, p. 44.

7. ibid.

8. See note 1 above.

9. ibid.

10. Committee on Infectious Diseases. *Report of the Committee on Infectious*

Diseases, 22nd ed., Elk Grove Village, Ill.: American Academy of Pediatrics, 1991.

11. See note 1 above.
12. www.cdc.gov/std/hpv.
13. ibid.
14. See note 3 above.

FIVE

1. John Graydon, "Depression." *University of Michigan Advances in Psychiatry Audiology Library* 30, no. 16 (2002).
2. Maurice Blackman, "Adolescent Depression" Originally published in *The Canadian Journal of CME*, May 1995. Available on-line. http:www.mentalhealth.com/mag1/p51-dp01.html.
3. Armand M. Nicholi, Jr., ed., *The Harvard Guide to Psychiatry*, 3rd ed. Cambridge, Mass.: The Belknap Press of Harvard University Press, 1999, pp. 622-623.
4. ibid.
5. A. M. Culp, M. M. Clyman, and R. E. Culp, "Adolescent Depressed Mood, Reports of Suicide Attempts, and Asking for Help." *Adolescence* 30 (1995): 827-837
6. See note 3 above, p. 623.
7. See note 5 above.
8. See note 3 above, p. 623.
9. Lydia A. Shrier, Sion Kim Harris, and William R. Beardslee, "Temporal Associations Between Depressive Symptoms and Self-reported Sexually Transmitted Disease Among Adolescents." *Archives of Pediatrics and Adolescent Medicine* 156 (2002): 599-606.
10. Kara Joyner and J. Richard Udry, "You Don't Bring Me Anything But Down: Adolescent Romance and Depression." *Journal of Health and Social Behavior* 41 (2000): 369-391.
11. Malcolm Ritter, "Teen Love Hurts; Falling In Love Makes Teens Prone to Depression and Alcohol Abuse." Internet on-line. www.abcnews.go.com/sections/living/DailyNews/teenlove010215.html.

12. See note 3 above, p. 619.

13. ibid.

SIX

1. S. J. Ventura, W. D. Mosher, S. C. Curtin, J. C. Abma, and S. Henshaw, *Trends in Pregnancies and Pregnancy Rates by Outcome: Estimates for the United States 1976-96*. National Center for Health Statistics, Centers for Disease Control and Prevention. Vital Health and Statistics Series no. 21 (56), 2000.

2. S. J. Ventura, W. D. Mosher, S. C. Curtin, J. C. Abma, and S. Henshaw, "Trends in Pregnancy Rates for the United States, 1976-97: An Update." National Vital Statistics Reports, vol. 49, no. 4. Hyattsville, Md.: National Center for Health Statistics, 2001.

3. ibid.

4. See note 1 above.

5. *Trends in Sexual Activity and Contraceptive Use Among Teens*, ChildTrends Research Brief. Internet on-line. www.childtrends.org/r_ac.asp.

6. ibid.

7. J. Abma, A. Chandra, W. Mosher, L. Peterson, and L. Piccinino, *Fertility, Family Planning and Women's Health: New Data from the 1995 National Survey of Family Growth*. National Center for Health Statistics, Centers for Disease Control and Prevention. Vital Health and Statistics Series no. 23 (19), 1997.

8. See note 5 above.

9. P. D. Darney, L. S. Callegari, A. Swift, E. S. Atkinson, and A. M. Robert, "Condom Practices of Urban Teens Using Norplant Contraceptive Implants, Oral Contraceptives, and Condoms for Contraception." *American Journal of Obstetrics and Gynecology* 180 (1999): 929-937.

SEVEN

1. "Condom Use by Adolescents (RE0059)." American Academy of Pediatrics Policy Statement. *Pediatrics* 107 (2001): 1463-1469.

2. ibid.

3. ibid.

4. www.niaid.nih.gov/dmid/stds/condomreport.pdf.

5. National Institute of Allergy and Infectious Diseases, National Institutes of Health, Department of Health and Human Services. *Workshop Summary: Scientific Evidence On Condom Effectiveness for Sexually Transmitted Disease Prevention*, July 20, 2001.

6. "Citing 'Failed Efforts' to Inform Public of Condom 'Ineffectiveness,' Physician Groups, Politicians Ask CDC Head to Resign." July 25, 2001. Daily HIV/AIDS Report, The Henry J. Kaiser Family Foundation (Kaisernetwork.org). Internet on-line. www.kaisernetwork.org/daily_reports/rep_index.cfm?hint=1&DR_ID=5980.

7. "Report Questions Condoms' Disease Prevention Ability," *Washington Post*, 20 July 2001, sec. A, p. A1.

8. "*Federal Panel on Condoms Offers Crucial Warnings to Sexually Active Americans, Says The Medical Institute for Sexual Health..*" NIH Condom Report Press Release. *Media Advisories*, Austin, Tex.: The Medical Institute for Sexual Health, July 19, 2001.

9. "Scientific Review Panel Confirms Condoms Are Effective Against HIV/AIDS, But Epidemiological Studies Are Insufficient for Other STDs." Press Release, H.H.S. News, U.S. Department of Health and Human Services, July 2001. Available at www.hhs.gov/news/press/2001pres/20010720.html.

10. See note 5 above.

11. Saifuddin Ahmed *et al.*, "HIV Incidence and Sexually Transmitted Disease Prevalence Associated with Condom Use: A Population Study in Rakai, Uganda." *AIDS* 15 (2001): 2171-2179

12. See note 8 above.

13. ibid.

14. A. Wald, A. G. M. Langenberg, K. Link, *et al.*, "Effect of Condoms on Reducing the Transmission of Herpes Simplex Virus Type 2 from Men to Women." *Journal of the American Medical Association* 285 (2001): 3100-3106.

15. See note 8 above.

16. See note 11 above.

17. Jared M. Baeten *et al.*, "Hormonal Contraception and Risk of Sexually Transmitted Disease: Results from a Prospective Study." *American Journal of Obstetrics and Gynecology* 183 (2001): 380-385.

18. See note 11 above.

19. See note 11 above.

20. L. Ku, F. L. Sonenstein, and J. H. Pleck, "The Dynamics of Young Men's Condom Use During and Across Relationships." *Family Planning Perspectives*. 26 (1994): 246-251.

21. See note 4 above.

22. G. Paz-Bailey *et al.*, "Condom Protection Against STD: A Study Among Adolescents Attending a Primary Care Clinic in Atlanta." Presented at the 2002 National STD Prevention Conference, San Diego, Calif., March 4-7, 2002. Abstract B9D.

23. See note 19 above.

24. ibid.

25. F. L. Sonenstein, L. Ku, L. C. F. Turner, and J. H. Pleck, "Changes in Sexual Behavior and Condom Use Among Teenaged Males: 1988 to 1995." *American Journal of Public Health* 88 (1998): 956-959.

26. L. Warner, J. Clay-Warner, J. Boles, and J. Williamson, "Assessing Condom Use Practices: Implications for Evaluating Method and User Effectiveness." *Sexually Transmitted Diseases* 25 (1998): 273-277.

27. ibid.

28. ibid.

29. R. A. Crosby and W. L. Yarber, "Perceived Versus Actual Knowledge About Correct Condom Use Among U.S. Adolescents: Results from a National Study," *Journal of Adolescent Health* 28 (2001): 415-420.

EIGHT

1. "Teens, Sex and the Media." Mediascope.org. Internet on-on-line. www.mediascope.org/pubs/ibriefs/tsm.htm.

2. P. G. Christenson and D. F. Roberts, *It's Not Only Rock & Roll.* Cresskill, N. J.: Hampton Press, 1998, p. 123.

3. ibid., pp. 142-143.

4. "Facts in Brief: Teen Sex and Pregnancy." (1998). *1995 National Survey of Family Growth and 1995 National Survey of Adolescent Males.* New York: The Alan Guttmacher Institute, 1998.

5. "New Study Finds Kids Spend Equivalent of Full Work Week Using Media." Press Release, November 29, 1999. Menlo Park, Calif.: The Henry J. Kaiser Family Foundation.

6. Dale Kunkel *et al.*, "Sex on TV: Content and Context. " A Biennial Report to the Kaiser Family Foundation. Menlo Park: Calif.: The Henry J. Kaiser Family Foundation, February 1999.

7. Miriam E. Bar-on, Danile D. Broughton, Susan Buttross, Suzanne Corrigan *et al.*, "Sex, Contraception, and the Media." *Pediatrics* 107 (2001): 191-194.

8. "More TV Shows Include Sexual Content; Safer Sex Message Most Common When Teen Characters or Sexual Intercourse Are Involved." Press Release, February 6, 2002. Menlo Park, Calif.: The Henry J. Kaiser Family Foundation.

9. "Teens, Sex and TV." Survey Snapshot. Kaiser Family Foundation. Publication #3229 April 2002. Internet on-line. www.kff.org.

10. See note 7 above.

11. See note 6 above.

12. "Children and the Internet." Mediascope.org. Internet on-line. www.mediascope.org/pubs/ibriefs/ci.htm.

13. See note 7 above.

14. Armand M. Nicholi, Jr., ed., *The Harvard Guide to Psychiatry*, Cambridge, Mass.: The Belknap Press of Harvard University Press, 1978.

15. Aletha C. Huston, Ellen Wartella, and Edward Donnerstein, "Measuring the Effects of Sexual Content in the Media." A Report to the Kaiser Family Foundation. Menlo Park: Calif.: The Henry J. Kaiser Family Foundation, May 1998.

NINE

1. R. B. Rothenberg *et al.*, "Using Social Network and Ethnographic Tools to Evaluate Syphilis Transmission." *Sexually Transmitted Diseases* 25 (1998): 154-160.

2. "The Lost Children of Rockdale County." From 1999 PBS Online and WGBH/FRONTLINE. Internet on-line. www.pbs.org/wgbh/pages/frontline/shows/georgia/new.

3. Sexuality Information and Education Council of the United States (SIECUS) "Non-Coital Behaviors That Put Teens at Risk for HIV and Other STDs." *SHOP Talk: School Health Opportunities and Progress Bulletin* 5, no. 22 (2001). Internet on-line. www.thebody.com/siecus/behaviors.html.

4. ibid.

5. "Safer Sex, Condoms, and 'the Pill.'" *Sexsmarts* (a public information publication), November 2000. Menlo Park, Calif.: The Henry J. Kaiser Family Foundation. Internet online. www.kff.org/content/2000/20001127a/SafeSexSummary.pdf

6. Lisa Remez, "Oral Sex Among Adolescents: Is It Sex or Is It Abstinence?" *Family Planning Perspectives* 32 (2000): 298-304.

7. ibid.

8. "Teens Say Oral Sex 'Doesn't Count' As More Engage." LifeDate, Family Life Issues. Internet on-line www.lutheransforlife.org/lifedate/2001/spring/teens_say_oral_sex_doesnt_count.html.

9. Oral Sex and STDs, Fact Sheet, Centers for Disease Control, Dec. 2000.

10. See note 6 above.

11. ibid.

12. "Lesbian, Gay, Bisexual and Transgendered, and Questioning Youth." *SIECUS Report* 29, no. 4, April/May (2001).

13. "When Kids Don't Have a Straight Answer" (Departments: Health and Fitness). *NEAToday Online* March 2001. Internet on-line. www.nea.org/neatoday/0103/.

14. R. Garofalo *et al.*, "The Association between Health Risk Behaviors

and Sexual orientation among a School-based Sample of Adolescents," *Pediatrics* 101 (1998): 895-902.

15. See note 13 above.

16. R. Garofalo, R. C. Wolf, L. S. Wissow, E. R. Woods, and E. Goodman. "Sexual Orientation and Risk of Suicide Attempts Among a Representative Sample of Youth." *Archives of Pediatric and Adolescent Medicine* 153 (1999): 487-493.

17. "Millions of Young People Mix Sex with Alcohol or Drugs—With Dangerous Consequences." Press Release, Feb. 6, 2002. Menlo Park, Calif.: The Henry J. Kaiser Family Foundation, in conjunction with The National Center on Addiction and Substance Abuse of Columbia University.

18. "Girl, 13, Killed by Man She Met Through Online Sex Chat Room." The Associated Press; May 22, 2002.

19. Barbarisi, D. "Ex-teacher Pleads Guilty in Internet Sex Case." *Providence (Rhode Island) Journal*, 19 June 2002, p. C-04.

TWELVE

1. *With One Voice: America's Adults and Teens Sound Off About Teen Pregnancy, A National Survey*. Washington, D.C.: The National Campaign to Prevent Teen Pregnancy, April 2001.

Index